Country Views

The Essential Agrarian Commentaries of Zachary Michael Jack

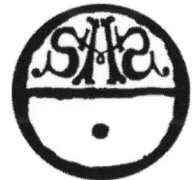

Tall Corn Books
Ice Cube Press, LLC
North Liberty, Iowa, USA

Country Views: The Essential Agrarian Commentaries of Zachary Michael Jack

Copyright © Zachary Michael Jack

First Edition

ISBN 9781948509169

Tall Corn Book, imprint of
Ice Cube Press, LLC (Est. 1991)
North Liberty, Iowa 52317
www.icecubepress.com | steve@icecubepress.com

All rights reserved.

No portion of this book may be reproduced in any way without permission, except for brief quotations for review, or educational work, in which case the publisher shall be provided copies. The views expressed in *Country Views* are solely those of the author, not the Ice Cube Press, LLC.

The paper used in this publication meets the minimum requirements of the American National Standard for Information Sciences—Permanence of Paper for Printed Library Materials, ANSI Z39.48-1992.

Manufactured in USA

For Steve,
with deepest gratitude
for the roots you sink
and the voices
you grow

Contents

Introducing *Country Views* 7

PART ONE: GROUNDWORK 13

    Portrait of a Harvest 15

    When High-Speed Internet Comes to the Slow Lane 19

    Beware the Fencer-in-Chief 23

    A Man among Marching Women 27

    Growing Seasons 30

    Cultivating a Country View 37

PART TWO: AXES TO GRIND 43

    Angling for Amazon 45

    In Praise of Barnyard English 49

    Last Man Standing 53

    We're Dying Here 56

    We Live and Die by Chemical Agriculture 61

    The Rural Health Care Crisis Is Real 65

    The Gift of Homecoming 68

    Rural Ghouls 72

    Cyber Monday in the Country 77

PART THREE: HOLIDAYS 81

    Holidays on Ice 83

    Christmas Wishes 86

    May Day 90

    Mothers' Day 93

Our Ancestors Sleep Down the Road 96

Father's Day and the Film That Gets
    Rural America Right 98

Agrarian Fireworks 102

PART FOUR: POLITICS 107

Breakaway Agrarian Republics 109

The Red Glow of Pyrotechnic Shifts 114

When the Government Says Go 118

New Crops and Old Worries 123

Savoring Straw Polls 127

The Plot of Grassroots Politics 130

Family Business Is Not Necessarily Nepotism 134

Political Epistles 137

Too Old to Rock and Roll, but Young
    Enough to Protest 143

Color Me Purple 146

PART FIVE: SEASONS 151

Moving Beyond "It Could Have Been Worse" 153

A New Diluvial Normal 155

Summer Whirls 158

Barefoot Eras 161

Skunk Hours 164

Seasonal Disaffections 166

Mind of Winter 170

February's Got Teeth 173

Time for Cheering 177

Twilight-time: An Open Letter 180

Rural Rip Van Winkle 184

Autumnal Swings 188

Afterword: A Look Back at *Country Views* 191

Acknowledgments 202

About the Author 205

Introducing *Country Views*

I began my career as an agrarian scholar-writer in 2001 with the good fortune of anthologizing and editing the work of the foremost agrarian educators of their day—Wendell Berry among them—in a first-of-its-kind agrarian anthology entitled *Black Earth and Ivory Tower: New American Essays from Farm and Classroom*. Though I was soon to return to the home farm in Iowa, at the time I was renting a tobacco farm in east Tennessee while commuting to a nearby small college to teach courses in Social Change and Service Learning. There the tobacco bust had already begun to do to Appalachian growers what the farm bust now threatens to do to commodity crop food producers in the Midwest and Great Plains. When I began renting in east Tennessee in 2001 tobacco was being grown on about 26,000 acres statewide. In Greene County, Tennessee, alone, tobacco occupied nearly 5000 acres.

Tobacco in Tennessee, and indeed throughout the Mid-South, had just begun a historic period of contraction in 1997 (a decade later in 2007 only about 4000 acres were being grown in all of east Tennessee and a mere 500 in all of Greene County), and yet agrarianism as a philosophy was alive and well in the Appalachians. On our small liberal arts campus community service and service learning—John Dewey's learning by doing—thrived. In the morning my students and I would gather together to study such subjects as Writing for Social Change and Civic Journalism; after lunch we would reconvene to put those and other classroom lessons to the test, volunteering for conservation work at national parks or advocacy work at local sustainable agriculture organizations. At night faculty and staff came together to hear spontaneous bluegrass jams played at rural crossroads markets and general stores. A few miles down the road in downtown Greeneville students and educators could visit the one-time capital of the Lost State of Franklin, a secessionist agrarian republic envisioned by egalitarian farmers and frontiersmen and women that had once vied to become America's fourteenth state.

Life in east Tennessee and western North Carolina in the late 1990s and early 2000s offered me a case study in agrarian living well beyond what I had known in my native Midwest. Though development was rapidly supplanting agriculture in east Tennessee and western North Carolina, agrarian values were, paradoxically, on the rise. Regionalism flourished, with a surfeit of new Appalachian-focused books, magazines, annuals, and academic conferences launched to help maintain and reclaim regional identity amid rapid gentrification and in-migration. I learned quickly that a yeoman's spirit often bloomed among ex-ruralites in whom the economic necessity of leaving the land had engendered a compensatory impulse to protect endangered folkways and heritages fondly recalled from childhood. Many former country dwellers could no longer live rurally themselves, but they were determined to make sure that the agrarian life remained a viable choice for others. Hence on-the-farm populations ebbed even as agrarian sentiments swelled.

Since my re-introduction to agrarianism in the foothills of east Tennessee I have continued to work the land while searching for a unified theory capable of infusing agrarian interests, folkways, and habits of mind into higher education, history, politics, media, and public policy. Indeed for all the completeness of my agricultural grounding, when I leave my small Midwestern farm to teach, to learn, and to share my experiences, I am continually amazed by the power of the agrarian mind to reinsert itself, finding relevance and resonance in corners where I hadn't thought to look. It's a mindset that bears continuous fruit, growing where it's least expected. At other times it lays fallow, a seed waiting for the right time to germinate.

In his 2015 essay "Farmland Without Farmers" Wendell Berry points out a much overlooked part of agrarianism: the pleasure it offers in growth and growing. His words are worth quoting:

> If people who live and work in the country don't also enjoy the country, a valuable and necessary part of life is missing.... There is pleasure in the work of maintenance, the redemption of things worn or broken, that must go on almost continuously. There is pleasure in the growing, preserving, cooking, and eating of the good food that the family's own land provides. But around this core of the life and work of the farm are clustered other pleasures, in their way also life-sustaining.

Just how to define the unique responsibilities, obligations, and pleasures of agrarianism challenges the rural mind. Maurice Telleen, for example, opens his essay "The Agrarian Mind-set" with a surprising admission: "I don't know quite how to skin this cat called agrarianism," and yet he goes on to fashion a remarkably cogent definition of the philosophy's esprit de corps.

Agrarianism, he argues, puts a "strong emphasis on personal behavior and its consequences—both long- and short-term—and even on eternal life. Eternal life, not as promise or reward for being 'good' or 'saved' but as an inescapable contract...." In a nutshell agrarianism is an ecology, the writer observes, adding, "We are born into a web of life that both precedes and follows us. Some of it is understood and some of it isn't.... Neutrality is not an option." After much soul-searching Telleen concludes, "What I think we can claim for agrarianism is that it is a central contract fashioned to work in a time and place.... Its job description is to function in such a way that it honors and maintains the earth, sustains and perpetuates community, shelters and benefits the citizens thereof, and respects the commonwealth for what it is: the common wealth.... It is more of a preservationist than a conqueror."

I like and respect this definition, in part because it demonstrates that agrarianism, like religion itself, can serve as a worldview, a value system, and a spiritual guide all at once. For me agrarianism offers a way of looking at the world—a country view—characterized by a healthy suspicion of groupthink, an emphasis on stewardship, cultivation, creativity, and higher learning, as well as a penchant for championing that which is near at hand—the local and the regional. To my mind agrarianism also recommends a healthy amount of prove-it-to me contrarianism, the sounding of all due cautionary notes, and a generous dose of humility and self-deprecation. As a mindset it's characteristically unwilling to settle for surfaces and superficialities, honoring the difficult over the expedient. In many ways it's a balky workhorse—inarguably powerful once moved, but maddeningly choosy in determining which master it serves. In a world increasingly characterized by painful shortages on one hand and gross excesses on the other, of extreme courage and brazen corruption, the agrarian mindset, with its cultivator's emphasis on sustainable growth, is needed now more than ever. Little wonder that its clarion call was heard in another era of conspicuous shortages and horrific transgressions: World War II.

In 1946 my great-grandfather, a Quaker-born advocate for chemical-free organic farming, digressed from his more serious chapters on soil science to argue for the basic goodness of rural life. In his book of that year, *The Furrow and Us*, he opines:

> Who can plant a seed in the ground, watch it sprout and grow and reproduce in abundance to feed a hungry world and not love the soil that mothered the seed? Who can walk barefoot in the freshly turned furrow as a youngster and not feel the thrill of it? Who can crumble the rich, black earth in their hands and not realize the preciousness of it to human life nor feel the excitement at all the mysteries it holds. Who fully realizes the high calling of farming and the possibilities it holds?

Across the generations his words remind we who are concerned with growth, with cultivation, with the mysteries of nature and its seasons, that when we nurture and cultivate we are all agrarians engaged in the yeoman's work, whether we hang our hat in the city or the country. In putting our collective shoulder to the difficult task of reinventing and re-sowing our democracy, we plant the seeds whose fruits future generations will surely reap.

Agrarianism aims to plow a new furrow in the long-standing distrust and misunderstanding of rural places inside of, and beyond, the halls of the world's colleges, universities, bureaucracies, and think-tanks, where too often that which is deeply rooted is viewed as willfully obstinate, contrarian, or backward—in short, an impediment to "progress" as defined by ruling elites and technocrats. Conversely, agrarian instigations, provocations, lamentations, appreciations, and benedictions— such country views as make up the book that follows—put the full breadth of a uniquely redeeming philosophy into varied practice. As Telleen enjoins, such advocacies are not neutral, nor do they aspire to be. The emphasis throughout is on the precious thing at the root of the agrarian worldview: growth. Individual growth, spiritual growth, community growth, cultural growth, intellectual growth—all leading, one hopes, to a better understanding and fuller flowering of the agrarian mind.

The commentaries, columns, and op-eds that follow reflect the sum of my agrarian thinking and writing over a ten-year period. The emphasis throughout is on the brevity expected of the editorial, op-ed, column, and commentary. Ranging from about six hundred words at their most concise to approximately fifteen hundred at their most developed, the pensees and provocations collected in *Country Views* aim for the deep, clean cut characteristic of both swords and plowshares. There is ground lovingly prepared here, as well as axes to grind, growing seasons both difficult and benign to negotiate, and holidays and other blessed occasions to celebrate in search of the fair yet formidable spirit that dwells in the hearts of those who seek to better appreciate country views.

Part I:
Groundwork

Portrait of a Harvest

Farming and caring for the land are far more subtle businesses than most care to realize, and to a fault farmers and land stewards aren't always given to explaining or justifying their methods.

This means that to appreciatively read the text and subtext of a growing season sometimes requires an almost ethnographic methodology, even for those of us still living on the land. Agriculture is a culture after all—full of enduring folkways and rapidly changing methods and mores. Like any culture it possesses its own sometimes Byzantine technologies, symbologies, and spiritualties.

Of all the small and subtle clues to farming's radically changed landscape perhaps the first and least obvious is the paucity of numbers. Folks from the coasts sometimes lump Corn Belt citizens together as "a bunch of farmers," or "salt of the earth types," but in real terms such farmers grow fewer by the year. According to the latest Agricultural Census only about 48,000 principal operators list farming as their primary occupation in the heart of the heartland: Iowa. If we crowded them all—at our peril of, course—into the University of Iowa's Kinnick Stadium on a single Big Ten football Saturday, more than 30 percent of the seats would still remain empty. The average age of principal operators (a whisker over 57 and aging) surprises, too, given the youthful face of small, sustainable, organic, specialized, and boutique agriculture. In rural Tennessee, where I began my career as an agrarian writer-scholar on a rented tobacco farm, the numbers aren't much better. There just over 79,000 principal operators work their acres statewide, a number that would only half fill NASCAR's famous shrine to speed, the Bristol Motor Speedway in Bristol, Tennessee.

Bear in mind that for many years the USDA has defined a farm "as any place that produced and sold, or normally would have sold, $1,000 or more of agricultural products during the Census year." If we live in a city, and have a rooftop garden or patio planted densely with a valuable crop grown for sale, we could be a farmer. Even if we only sold $150 this year due to weather, or insect plague, or, in theory, any life event that prevented us from realizing the full financial potential of our crop, we still may be a farmer on "points," according to the USDA system. Of course here it is important to note, according to Farm Policy Facts, that the 210,000 farmers nationally with sales of more than $250,000 produce 80 percent of the country's food and fiber.

A farmer is a difficult thing to count precisely because he or she doesn't always care to be counted, perhaps explaining why the USDA is so keen to include just about any food- or fiber-producing operation in their once-every-five-years bean-counting. Visit the department's website and you'll be exhorted to "Make Sure Your Farm or Ranch Counts!" Large or small, the bureaucracy notes, "your agricultural operation is important.... This includes retirement/lifestyle farms and ranches that grow a small amount of plants or crops or keep only a few animals, up to the largest of operations.... Landowners that only have income from government programs are also counted as farms."

It's a difficult profession to isolate and pin down, too, for the jack-of-all-trades virtuosity it requires. In this postmodern age, and more and more, a farmer is as a farmer does. In Iowa, the heart of the heartland by any measure, nearly 40 percent of those listed as farm operators report working more than two hundred days each year off the farm. Of the 89,000 or so individual farms counted there, nearly 20 percent total less than 100 acres.

I had begun this piece with the intention of offering a more impressionistic take on harvest time, my favorite of all seasons, as it is for many farm- and food-loving people. I had wanted to write a dispatch touching on all the little things that have changed in farming since I was a teenager—for instance the fact that in the days before early-maturing soybeans we always put the corn head on our combine first; or how, in east Tennessee, the collapse of the quota system and price supports for tobacco farmers mean that in some counties where tobacco once ruled as king it now occupies less than 500 acres total.

Agriculture depends more than ever on technology, and, as in most professions, if you're not out on the front lines armed with the latest and greatest, you're a dinosaur. What I do know is that the commodity crop farming happening all around us deserves a much closer read than most non-rural citizens are willing to give it. I know, too, that because reading about necrotic soybeans and their sudden death syndromes or the slow death of the tobacco industry in Kentucky is something less than a page-turner for many metropolitans, most network TV stations and newspapers even in farm country long ago axed their ag-dedicated reporters and broadcasters.

Old-timers, ex-farmers, and born-on-the-farmers are wont to talk about these subtle yet transformative changes in agriculture; many privately squirrel away the artifactual evidence of when farming changed beyond their recognition. My father always said that when the average man or woman on the streets couldn't tell you, within twenty-five cents, what the price of corn was on any given day, it had ceased to be an agricultural state, and rue the day. Another farm-reared friend claims that moment happened when hay bales grew too large for a single person to lift.

Whatever your own private beliefs about contemporary agriculture, it's worth remembering each and every harvest season that large-scale farmers and food-producers are not the insensate, unsubtle, imperceptive businessmen they're often made out to be. I'll bet, in fact, that they spend more time thinking about us, worrying over us, and puzzling over us—our inscrutable and sometimes volatile changes in taste and temperament—than we do about them.

When High-Speed Internet Comes to the Slow Lane

One day last summer a convoy of trucks from the local utility barreled up my long lonesome rural lane bearing jubilant word that they had brought the world to my doorstep—their words, not mine—via the wonders of high-speed internet. They descended like locusts, without warning, and with, as the generals say, overwhelming force.

I'll admit that initially I was suspicious of their sudden display of interest; as any rural landowner knows utility companies challenge private property rights in often uncomfortable ways. They enjoy easements up and down even the most forsaken rural drive, and even though smart-meters have largely replaced meter-readers, the utility folks, like in-laws, insist on visiting when and how often they like.

Still, as their trenchant trenching commenced that day, and the hole carrying the fiber optic cable churned its inexorable way up my drive like a righteous mole, I couldn't help but be flattered by their attentions; those of us who live on farms beyond a forty-five-minute drive from the nearest metropolis are accustomed to being ignored where public works are concerned.

Often we thank our lucky stars that we exist beyond the purview of the overreaching, overweening utility barons and DOT overlords, but it's also nice to have an occasional bone thrown our way. You see, we're used to being a low priority in the increasingly desperate fiscal triage strategies adopted by state, county, and local government, to say nothing of private enterprise. It's an economy of scale, we're given to understand; there are so few of us here of the ideal discretionary spending profile that in a condition of scarcity we're all too willing to wait our turn in the interests of the common good.

Just down the road stand electrical poles dating back to the original rural electrification of the 1940s—twisted, gnarled, cedar erections that look palpably more like tree than post, strung with wire and the sort of glass insulators that fetch a pretty penny in urban antique and curio shops where they are associated, ironically, with the long-ago. My land-line still pops and crackles with the not-unpleasing "noise" of the sort that lately caused Verizon to settle with the Feds for $5 million in penalties for allegedly offering substandard and unreliable land-line service to its rural customers.

Not long ago The Boston Consulting Group (BGG) came out with polling data documenting what consumers living in industrialized G-20 nations worldwide would be willing to go without before they would give up the internet. 70 to 80 percent, the group found, would consistently forsake staples and social lubricants such as alcohol and coffee for a joy-ride on the information superhighway. Nearly a quarter in the United States would sacrifice sex compared to more than half of those surveyed in Japan, who would gladly pass over the prospect of a little hanky-panky for a little clicky-clicky.

I suspect had the Boston survey wonks paid closer attention to rural Americans they would have uncovered dramatically different priorities. I know plenty of farm neighbors, for instance, who prize their morning Folgers or Yuban above all else, and ditto the sacred, farm-enabling bond of fertility shared with partner or spouse. They would no doubt see in the urban-biased data the solipsism of a distracted people they would claim are going to hell in a handbasket—a people who would rather surf the internet than steal a kiss beneath the sheets or wrest a living from a frustratingly uncooperative and analog earth. It's not a simple equation, I'll grant you (I can think of neighbors, too, who would gladly ditch the quittin'-time Miller Lite for a nightly swill of the internet), but they are in the minority. However, this too seems destined to change as the laying of new cable brings internet-dependent out-migrators into the hinterlands the way the way rail lines of the nineteenth century carried urbanites west.

As a consequence of generations of doing without the niceties and fineries of urban life, many older ruralites have developed a compensatory we-can-get-along-without-it, thank-you-very-much attitude toward new technologies. As my sister and I came of age in the 1970s and early 1980s, for instance, my rural family did without the cable television we both secretly longed for and outwardly decried. (We occasionally conned our aunts and uncles in town into videotaping HBO and Showtime movies for their country cousins.)

Later, I made do with AOL dial-up for years until one day the modem unexpectedly refused to make the requisite digital handshake, and a customer service agent in India informed me AOL had canceled its service in my rural area—not enough interest. Thereafter I hung a cell signal-enabled USB internet device precariously out my living room window, shutting the sash down tightly on the cord while the device blinked cool blue until the snow falling outside the window covered its LED, and the thing would have to be brought inside like a farm dog needing warming up.

Given our proud history of country workarounds the day the high-speed cable tunneled its way up my lane and into my house produced, I admit, an almost erotic brand of pleasure. How had they guessed my secret yearnings? How could they possibly have found me here deep in my private wanting? No matter that the contractors hired to trench the lines knocked over my mailbox… they had actually come.

Like the long-forgotten country widower I was simply pleased that someone had remembered me. It didn't matter what they were hawking; I smiled, thanked them for coming, and bought some of what the nice young men were selling. There would be time later to ponder the consequences.

Beware the Fencer-in-Chief

Robert Frost's adage "good fences make good neighbors" enjoys the weight of papal decree where I grew up. Fences loom large in the agrarian psyche, describing to us and to others the size and shape of our dominion.

Now, one hundred and sixty-five years after my ancestors bought our land from homesteader David Platner, the cedar and barbed-wire erections that mark our territory serve little practical purpose, existing mostly as a remnant of bygone days when livestock rather than commodity crops ruled our world. Like cornerstones they remind us of the hard-won battles we've fought to make these acres our own and to protect them from endless cycles of debt, drought, disease, and pestilence. Their effect is mostly symbolic—like a family coat of arms in a clan that has long since given up swords for plowshares.

Little wonder, then, that when the time came for me to begin making decisions about our acres my mind turned to fences. I knew the aesthetics would improve without them, offering a clearer and less divided view of the fruitful land in which we had sunk our roots. The narrow strip of fence-line between me and my most immediate neighbor to the south had for some time stood as a de facto no man's land of waist-high weeds. Too tight a space to mow with the tractor and beyond the reach of herbicides it served as a visual reminder of the uneasy truce that pervades most lands located betwixt and between.

Once I made the mistake of trying to beautify this between-land by transplanting a handful of silver maples along its full width and breadth, hoping to turn the forlorn strip into a wildlife corridor. A week after I had finished the hard work of transplanting my neighbor tacked an indignant note to the door, arguing that the saplings would one day shade his corn. It seemed not to matter that the trees were set many yards back from our shared property line, or that by the time their canopy grew to the sun-blocking, yield-reducing proportions he imagined, we would both be dead. He wanted the saplings removed, posthaste, and I complied. And for a time an uneasy status quo returned to our borderlands.

My neighbor's objections must have been at least as much symbolic as they were practical. Whether fashioned from posts or from trees a fence suggests that the fencer has something worth keeping—something a neighbor might covet. A fence asserts an asymmetry of value. In rare cases where neighbors erect fences simultaneously, or share in the expense, the fence can indeed be a balm and cure. More often than not, however, the decision to build a wall is a unilateral one resulting from one party's desire to protect and preserve something the other party does not now possess but just as assuredly wants. Once erected it serves to remind the disinherited of their lack.

I had only hoped to find a place for the many maple saplings that had proliferated elsewhere on the farm, and transplanting them nearer the edge of the property saved me the trouble of mowing around them. A prosperous farmer, my neighbor certainly didn't need to exercise dominion over that narrow strip of borderland. And in sowing new trees where they hadn't been before I had begun a conversation in which he was determined to have the final word. After the vegetative fence came down, the Cold War between us as neighbors lasted until the following harvest, when I crossed over to his side to lend a hand.

Since that first across-the-fence encounter I've grown circumspect about the human desire to wall off what is ours from what is theirs. Far from making good neighbors, the building of a new fence exacerbates rather than mitigates conflict. So it is that across rural America landowners like me are ripping out the old barbed wire fences that section off our fields. In many cases we're tearing down the very barriers our ancestors put up to prevent cattle from roaming the open range.

Why take down a fence? Because as farmers and ranchers understand better than most, economies are fluid: the barbed wire that once served to keep out livestock grows obsolete in an era when cash crops rule. Fences may feel permanent, but economies and cultures exist in perpetual flux. And in a volatile global economy ruled by volatile leaders the fences we erect today to protect our assets are often those that limit our potential tomorrow.

In over twenty years of fence-building across a broad swath of rural America I've learned that fences come with a built-in paradox. While they make it difficult to get in, they make it proportionally difficult to get out. On Western ranches I've put up hundreds of feet of fence in ruggedly beautiful country. And with each post sunk I've experienced a sinking feeling at the logic of willingly sacrificing the long view for the myopic and often mythic protections of a wall.

Consider, too, this inconvenient truth: fences require perpetual maintenance. Like the fraught decision to apply a first coat of paint to a house, the building of a fence commits the Fencer, or in this case the Fencing Nation, to years of upkeep. Shouldn't risk-adverse don't-tread-on-me types like me—those of us predisposed to the fencer's mentality in the first place—be naturally wary of the no-horizon clause and no easy-out commitment of a permanent wall? Even the urbanite putting up store-bought fence panels from the local big-box store knows the frustration at having to "go around" where once they exited freely at their own convenience. It's a straight-up paradox: in fencing others out we often unwittingly box ourselves in.

Don't get me wrong: years of fence-building and mending have shown me that walls do indeed serve a purpose, though they are far from the uncomplicated cure-all politicians and policymakers would have us believe. Used strategically and with care they sometimes solve persistent problems between neighbors locked in territorial disputes or culture wars.

However, a fencing people and a fencing nation ought to be cautious where the impulse to cordon off is concerned. We should weigh carefully our own motives, the alleged benefits, and, most urgently, the literal and figurative cost of building walls the angels of our better natures might soon tear down.

A Man among Marching Women

Lately I've come to realize just how much my life has been moved by brave rural women activists. Sure, I've spent the last several years researching suffragette "General" Rosalie Gardiner Jones and the historic marches of her equal rights women's armies, but my time among marching women didn't begin with Jones, or in the many years I've spent teaching gender-related issues in college classrooms, or even in the lead-up to the Women's March on Washington. It began with a long-ago Fourth of July parade held deep in the countryside.

In 1986 the annual Independence Day parade in our local unincorporated river town of Cedar Bluff, Iowa, made national news. Even then our backwater Mardi Gras had a reputation for, as the *Daily Iowan* put it, "attracting odd and politically-oriented displays." Still, the Fourth of July events in Cedar Bluff were mostly a best-kept secret until 1986, when five women dressed as Lady Liberty rode topless on a women's rights float, making a statement against pornography and objectification of women's bodies. "Independence Day is an ideal time for our protest," Melissa Farley, one of the day's "bare-breasted women," told the world in a national UPI newswire story. There appeared to be no enforceable county ordinance to stop the display, county sheriff George Miller informed the national press corps, adding, "I don't believe there's a law that really prohibits it (nudity)."

I remember how anomalously adult I felt that day as a boy of twelve trusted by my mother and grandmother and aunts to witness the topless protest. At twelve I had never seen any woman's uncovered bosom other than my mother's, but I had been raised into tolerance by a long line of brave, sometimes brazen, farm women. For the Bicentennial parade in 1976 my own circle of women warriors, led by my mother and grandmother and aunts, dressed us boys as redcoats and revolutionaries and loaded us atop a parade float they'd hammered into life with their own hands. Breast-baring and stars-and-bars would seem strange bedfellows, but in 1976 they mingled freely in the rural Midwest and elsewhere. On television Lynda Carter's Wonder Woman costume represented a purposeful hybrid of the Amazon woman warrior of antiquity—tiara, modified breastplate, bracelets, and boots—and Lady Columbia, the long-standing female personification of America that predated the male Uncle Sam by at least a century.

Although his hands were tied our county sheriff clearly wished the shirtless women marchers might take their protest out of his otherwise peaceful agrarian county in 1986, when the Lady Liberties drew, according to a report from another national wire service, both "cheers and jeers" from spectators on hand to watch them ride across the bridge over the turbulent Cedar River. The *Daily Iowan* numbered the unruly crowd of spectators that day at approximately fifteen thousand in a river settlement that typically counted under fifty residents. One man "charged at Farley," according to a report, only to be restrained by one of the float's retinue of muscular male escorts—the "men's auxiliary," they called themselves.

What was it about the sight of women baring and braving it all for social justice that seemed to so unnerve our rural community? And whatever it was, I wonder if the fear will be the same or similar the next time women march on the National Mall, as it was in 1913, when a peaceful protest march made up of an estimated ten thousand women paraded up Pennsylvania Avenue to meet violence from angry male mobs. The violence against the armies led by Rosalie Gardiner Jones and Inez Milholland in 1913 (the later sporting a cape and riding atop not a parade float but a white horse like the Scythian woman warriors of old) resulted in an eleven-day Congressional inquiry and, ultimately helped pave the way for the ratification of the 19th Amendment granting women the right to vote.

Now, more than four decades after TV's Wonder Woman first drained the swamp and beat the bad guys in Washington DC, and a generation after a handful of women dared to march topless for their beliefs in Cedar Bluff, Iowa, some of my own students have begun packing their bags and arranging their rides to the latest Women's March on Washington. Meanwhile, I'm traveling across the Midwest sharing the forgotten story of "General" Jones's all-woman army of 1912 and 1913. And at every school and library at which I stop, there's a powerful moment when I recall how fortunate I am for the times that brave women have marched into my life and moved me to action.

Growing Seasons

Recently I found myself at the confluence of two tasks needing doing: one agricultural and the other bibliographic, the two, as agrarian writer Liberty Hyde Bailey knew best, not so very different in the end. The first was how to stave off the invasion of wild burdock and dandelion that found me, Hamlet-like, posing the to-weed-or-not-to-weed question. Should I strike out against the burdock and, by opposing, end it, or simply suffer the slings and arrows of its outrageous existence? That practical yeoman's dilemma mixed and mingled in my mind with the reading and reviewing of John Stempien's and John Linstrom's anthology *The Liberty Hyde Bailey Gardener's Companion*. Faced with acres of impressively elephantine burdock volunteering in every corner of the farmyard, my mind turned naturally to Bailey, who once wrote of this otherwise verboten species: "If a person wants to show his skill, he may choose the balky plant: but if he wants fun and comfort…he had better choose the willing one."

Nothing is more willing than wild burdock.

A long-time professor of experimental horticulture at Cornell University, Bailey championed the virtues of the much maligned burdock and the pesky dandelion throughout an oeuvre numbered at more than sixty-five books and more than a thousand articles. Throughout, he takes up the cause of weeds and other wayfaring and unwanted botanical strangers, so much so that his sympathies, farmers of his era felt, must surely have lain with the devil. Like naturalists John Muir, John Burroughs, and Henry David Thoreau before him, Bailey didn't see weeds as emblems of devilry, but as simple and unavoidable facts whose purpose and meaning the horticulturalist should work to divine.

"We are apt to covet the things which we cannot have; but we are happier when we love the things which grow because they must," Bailey wrote in his essay "General Advice," adding, "The man who worries morning and night about dandelions in the lawn will find great relief in loving the dandelions." A thoroughgoing sentimentalist, Bailey elsewhere waxes nostalgic about the dandelions of his long-ago boyhood on the farm, writing: "We hated them because we had made up our minds not to have them, not because they were unlovable…. Then if we must have them, we decided to love them. Where once were weeds are now golden coins scattered in the sun, and bees reveling in color, and we are happy!" It's his child-like exuberance, tempered with his scholar's circumspection, that makes Bailey such an important figure for a new generation of agrarians to know.

Like Bailey, I grew up on a Midwestern farm where loving a weed was a sin. I learned early on that how one regards a weed depends very much on one's perspective. To a true farmer, loving a weed—any weed—is to admit God's fallibility. To knowingly spare a weed in the field is to give an inch to nature's dominion, like refusing to trap the first of the mice slowly but surely wrecking the home. To begin to love the weed, or even to concede its existence, is a worldview the commodity food producer cannot allow himself if he wants to call himself a farmer, no less than a commanding general can allow himself sympathy with the enemy it is his sworn duty to defeat.

The town-dweller, by contrast, can be magnanimous in giving safe quarter to the willing volunteers growing wild behind the garage or in the basement window well. The wild burdock represents no real and present danger to the happy homeowner's carefully controlled lawn. Hemmed in by verdant nitrogen-fed bluegrass, here the weed is invited to be a welcome exotic, a happy accident of fate whose novelty the town-dweller is prepared to entertain for a season or two before wearying of it. For the farmer the same whimsical burdock is an existential threat. While the happy homeowner's patch amounts to perhaps ten square feet of benign neglect the farmer's 100-acre field represents over four million square feet of opportunity for the opportunistic invader to root down. Wild burdock gone to seed on such an epic scale is the stuff of yeoman's nightmares, like falling behind on the milking or the mowing, multiplied a hundredfold. And in farm and ranch country to fall behind on one's mowing is a sure sign of moral decline, like shopping for groceries in one's pajamas because one can't be bothered to put on pants.

If a weed was to be loved, it was the farmer's wife who would love it, and all of creation. Defending the right of a pigweed, cocklebur, or bindweed to exist threatened to emasculate the plowman, making him the object of ridicule or at least scandalous rumor among neighbors. In our barnyard my grandmother performed the part of patron saint of weeds by playing good cop to my grandfather's bad cop where unwanted plants were concerned. While my grandfather spent his mornings with a hand-held sprayer filled with herbicide, dead set against the idea that our barnyard should be anything but pristine, my grandmother gloried in the waist-high Queen Anne's lace that shot up between the cracks of the sunken concrete patio she claimed as her own. She loved wildness for its own sake, and adored it all the more for the bright contrast it offered between herself and her husband. Once emboldened, the umbrella of her amnesty soon extended to the glorious profusion of ditch weeds across the gravel road, where she would defiantly plant "Do Not Spray" signs in the weeks before the county would initiate its perennially wrong-headed efforts at weed-control.

It may have been the subversive in me, or simply the boy charmed by his raven-haired grandmother's contrarianism and charisma, but I too learned early on to love the weed as an emblem of all that my perfectionist father and grandfather disproved of. I found amusement in the heated arguments at the dinner table over whether this or that patch of hemlock or wild mustard should be allowed to live, predictably siding with Our Lady of Weeds, though in my naiveté I understood little then of the full import of the debate. Because my father's and grandfather's ongoing vigilance ensured that I never had to experience the horror of a once prosperous farm completely gone to seed, it was easy for me to view them as caricatures comical in their extremes. When it came to invasive species the men were villains, while my grandmother was a savior.

Only later, when it was my turn to steward the land, did I arrive at a more mindful middle ground, reconsidering both my grandmother's sainthood and my fathers' seeming devilry. I realized that my grandmother and I had something in common beyond our perverse desire to make life difficult for the Type-A men in our lives; we'd been afforded the position of critics because we had been spared any real responsibility for the upkeep and cultivation of the farm. Neither of us understood that the land, if uncultivated, did not magically return to Edenic tallgrass prairie.

When I began to take over the care of my own farm acres, my father gradually began to confess his sins to me. An award-winning conservation farmer and the grandson of pioneering organics advocate and author Walter Thomas Jack, he admitted that he considered spraying an absolute abomination, and that it pained him ethically, morally, and philosophically. He sprayed his crops, he said, because with my sister and me in school, and my grandfather nearing retirement, a tank full of Round-up or 2,4-D was a weapon of mass destruction he felt compelled to use in a war of absolute attrition that, for our continued livelihood, he had no choice but to win. 128 fluid ounces of herbicide could magically substitute for the labor of an entire family AWOL in town.

As if to absolve himself of the guilt he felt over his sparing use of chemicals, late in life he relayed to me a traumatic memory that had lodged itself deep in his psyche. The memory concerns him and my grandfather alone with garden hoes in a hundred-acre field choked with morning glories. He never forgot how frightened he was, a boy barely old enough to attend elementary school, forced to witness his own father's fear at the desperate odds they faced. It was the two of them, alone at war, against tens of thousands of invaders threatening to ruin their crop and the work of five generations. Until his dying day my father wept openly every time he told the story.

In the twenty-first century it has become fashionable for rural sons and daughters to feel as if they have transcended the sins of their mothers and fathers. Maybe their mother smoked, but they have never so much as inhaled. Perhaps their meat-and-potatoes-loving father died of a massive heart attack at fifty-five, but they obsessively watch their cholesterol and eat right; he never took a day off work in his life, but they take three weeks of paid vacation. And yet just because we wear khakis to work instead of pinstripe overalls, and have traveled around the world instead of just to the state capital, does not mean we are morally superior.

After leaving home in South Haven, Michigan, Liberty Hyde Bailey transformed from farm boy to Ivy League scholar, exemplifying the pattern of increasing educational attainment and upward mobility that most in the twenty-first century equate with that chimera called success. Raised in a yeoman family that hated weeds as creed, Bailey learned as an adult to celebrate the verboten burdock, unappreciated dandelion, and "lusty pigweed," among other undesirables. He spent his career in a classroom teaching Cornell University students to respect the genius for survival inherent in the very plants his farming forebears fought bitterly to mow, kill, or otherwise plow under.

My own life pattern, and the pattern of many farm-reared children, is similar to Bailey's, though I do not call it transcendence. I've learned from maintaining my own land to first trust the opinion of experts like Bailey who have lived the question and fought the battles about which others merely speculate. I know why it is that the general who has been to war best understands the value of peace.

In the end I fall on my grandmother's and great-grandfather's side of the family tree when it comes to resisting the ravages of chemical-intensive farming, and more so for having faced a field of weeds too prolific to control by mechanical means alone. I believe in the wisdom of rising generations that say no to chemicals and yes to organics and sustainable living. But I wish to every one of agriculture's critics would fall the responsibility of managing a farm, market garden, or acreage, if only to better understand that the choice of whether to spray is something less than the black-and-white, good-and-evil conundrum it is made out to be. Real enlightenment comes from making informed choices, and informed choices come from practical hands-on experience with the options from which one is choosing.

On days when I wear my pleated pants to the office I slip all too easily into the role of critic, expertly honing in on the flaws inherent in others' choices. But on days when I don my father's clothes, and head out into a barnyard that threatens to overwhelm me with its fertility and its mysteries, the intellectual, philosophical, ethical certainties of my deskbound existence quickly evaporate. I'm left humbled not only by the loneliness and difficulty of the hands-on labor so few want to undertake anymore, but of the grayness of the options left me in a field full of wonder, and choices.

Cultivating a Country View

Not long ago an ominous headline came across my newsfeed as I sat down to breakfast to consider the day of haymaking and teaching ahead of me: "The Next American Farm Bust Is Upon Us." And yet lost in the misleading doom and gloom reporting of rural events in the nation's most metropolitan newspapers, then as now, is the remarkable endurance of agrarian values in a world where paradoxically fewer and fewer of us make our sole living working the land.

The *Wall Street Journal* article warned that for the first time since the Louisiana Purchase there would soon be fewer than two million farms in America, and yet even that statistic, sobering as it was, failed to convey agriculture's abiding influence on American culture. The well-meaning report, bylined Ransom, Kansas, neglected to mention that fully 80 percent of all rented farmland is owned by non-farming landlords, and many of these non-farming landlords were themselves born or raised on farms or in small farming communities. As these same aging landlords leave their land to the next generation over the next two decades, 70 percent of the nation's private farm and ranchland is expected to change hands in a cultural moment ripe with opportunity for renewal in the next generation.

That the land's new owners and stewards be versed in a philosophy—agrarianism—that has well-served landowners, landholders, land stewards, and legislators for centuries is best regarded as a national priority. In fact, the overall decline in farm population masks the deeper gains agrarianism has made in popular culture since my father was born on our then ninety-six-year-old family farm in 1950. In 1950 five million farms graced America, accounting for a total farm population of twenty-five million strong. Now, as so many in my father's age cohort—tens of millions of farm-reared Boomers—near retirement in non-farm professions, they return, in heart and in mind, to abiding wisdoms gleaned from childhoods lived on the land. Boomers who as young professionals carried their agrarian wisdoms and worldviews with them into the urban and suburban workplaces now stand poised to reclaim and reinvent them in retirement. Meanwhile, a burgeoning interest in Place Studies among students at colleges and universities yields new academic programs in the subject at such venerable institutions as the University of Iowa, the University of Nebraska, and my own North Central College, to name just a few.

A generation later, when I was born to our 500-acre, multi-generational Century Farm, the on-the-farm population had slipped to just under ten million despite the overall farm prosperity of the early and mid 1970s. More efficient than ever, farmers now accounted for just under five percent of the American labor force. Eighteen years later, when I graduated from high school, that percentage dropped to around 2.5 percent, while the overall farm population nationally declined to just under three million. But while the on-farm population dropped more than twenty million from my father's birth in 1950 to the last year such data was kept in the year 2000, the popularity of agrarian values soared among urbanites and suburbanites, many of whom had enjoyed rural or exurban upbringings a generation or two earlier. Others, new to the agrarian mindset, are buying organic, shopping local and regional, DIYing, "homesteading," slow-fooding, local or homeschooling—in short enacting core agrarian principles. While the total on-the-farm population dropped perilously close to three million by the year 2000, the rural non-farm population rose from a reported 45.6 million in 1970 to a 56.1 million in 2000. In short, while many families left the occupation of farming they did not leave rural living behind. Overall some seventy million North Americans are still classified as rural, a number that does not include the many tens of millions living in the small towns the US Census Bureau terms micropolitan areas.

As America grows increasingly suburban and urban, agrarians, whether they live in the city or in the country, too often find their values overlooked or ignored by many of the institutions the rural and small-town *demos* helped build—county and state government, colleges and universities, and the fourth estate made up of members of the national media, to name just a few. Concurrently, while chemical-intensive, large-scale commodity farming remains a national bogeyman for some, interest in shopping locally, living sustainably, and enacting a do-it-yourself lifestyle has spiked among young professionals eager to imagine their way out of the orthodoxies of urban and suburban life.

Contemporary agrarians understand that their stock periodically rises and falls in the eyes of the powerbrokers around them, whether those stakeholders are in government, higher education, or public policy. They know how quickly today's headlong rush toward urbanity might give way to yet another back-to-the-land movement. Even more acutely the agrarian understands that their way of life must be better and more energetically articulated to a generation of reader-consumers whose loyalties have been shaped by the ubiquities and homogeneities of suburban and urban upbringings. By analogy, if one has never tasted a tart, slightly bitter farm apple picked fresh from the orchard, how does one know to look beyond the preternatural, perfectly unsustainable Red Delicious on offer at the nearest grocery store? In a consumer-driven world where choice is limited in advance by invisible gatekeepers, we inevitably fill our carts with end-cap, eye-level items pre-arranged to draw our eye and our discretionary dollars. In attending to the socioeconomic disparities felt by rural and small-town communities, colleges, universities, and other nonprofits, think-tanks and advocacy groups must take up the challenge of educating consumers in a world where the items up for purchase are not just apples or oranges, but the ZIP codes where we live our lives, pay our taxes, and educate our children.

What would it take for tomorrow's professors, pedagogues, policymakers, and not-for-profit powerbrokers to cultivate a country view of the world around them? Place-based education, ardent localism and regionalism, experiential education, and community-engaged learning plant seeds sure to bear fruit in the future. Colleges and universities can help open minds to the idea that one's place is more than incidental or circumstantial, more than a place to land during a brief educational or professional stint, more than mere crash pad or launch pad for career ambitions, more than where one receives one's mail and cashes one's paycheck. In the rush toward more cosmopolitan living, preservation of the agrarian mind and the country views that mind honors and maintains should be as elemental and integral to democratic pluralism as a spirited defense of endangered ecologies.

Part II:
Axes to Grind

Angling for Amazon

John, a fellow ruralite, claims that we should thank our lucky stars that many of our Great Plains states were spared the frenzied competition to host Amazon.com's second global headquarters. The corporate bigwigs there, he claims, are all about what he calls a "Left Coast mentality." "Just look at what the Californication of Colorado, Nevada, and Idaho has already done," he insists, suggesting that the unquestioning acceptance of Amazon's creed is part of the deal it's hoping to strike with the host of its coveted headquarters. Amazon, John believes, would never find the urban progressivism it seeks in Wyoming's or South Dakota's native agrarianism, for example, but it would demand that its host state conform to its political views in the typical my-way-or-the-highway fashion of corporate bullies.

It's no secret that Amazon's CEO is a champion of urbanist and Blue State values, and the sweepstakes for his company's new North American HQ2 headquarters reflects its CEO's political predisposition. Corporate headquarters claims to need loads of affordable housing for a diverse workforce numbering in the tens of thousands, proximity to major highways, ready access to airports, and nearness to a major university. Predictably, the choices for the surprise "split" headquarters—New York City and the greater Washington DC/Northern Virginia metro—look very much like the ubiquitous "best cities to live in" and "smart cities" picks that too often reinforce the idea that urban and progressive is the sole recipe for quality of life.

As an educated seventh generation ruralite from deep in flyover country, and one who has been an Amazon Prime member for many years, I would like to ask Amazon to give rural America a fairer trial. Of the seven states who reportedly opted out of the Amazon sweepstakes, four—Montana, North Dakota, South Dakota, and Wyoming, are among the most rural and Republican—in other words, not Amazon-friendly territory at first glance. And yet a 2011 report by the U.S. Chamber of Commerce ranks three of those states (North Dakota, Wyoming, and South Dakota) among the top five growth performers nationwide.

Could Amazon ever see fit to headquarter itself in a rural ranching or mining state, provided that state met their logistical wish list, and, if not, why not? Are the Great Plains and northern Rocky Mountain states poorly run or economically unsound? Hardly. In fact, according to a 2016 study reported in *USA Today*, Amazon hold-out North Dakota topped the list of best-governed states, with Wyoming coming in at number four. According to the latest Bankrate.com figures, Montana, North Dakota, and South Dakota continue to boast the lowest foreclosure ratings in the nation, a calling card that speaks not just to their affordable housing, but to their fiscal discipline and ultimate economic stability.

To those on the coasts rural America's refusal to jump on the Amazon bandwagon may appear stubbornly self-defeating, fear-based, or even jingoistic or xenophobic—not worthy, in any case, of a high-minded corporation. But viewed in a more sympathetic light their rationale for withholding a bid might reasonably be interpreted as old-fashioned horse sense and an unwillingness to buy, with tax incentives and other costly giveaways, a golden ticket for a corporate lottery odds say they have little chance of winning despite affordable housing, ample land for warehousing, and often excellent and underused transportation networks.

Changing for others' sakes, chasing after the latest fad, or inflating the latest bubble has never been the modus operandi in places like Missoula or Cheyenne. By contrast Stonecrest, Georgia, in suburban Atlanta, reportedly offered to change its name to "Amazon" if the company headquartered within its city limits. Laissez-faire capitalists and free enterprisers would eagerly concede that Amazon has the right to choose with whom it associates—in this case opting for hypereducated, urbane, and highly mobile over the semi-rural and rooted. But in choosing for its new headquarters two of America's already well-endowed major metros, the internet commerce giant misses the vast swath of flyover country where populations, albeit small, are well-known for their willingness to work. And if Montana, Wyoming, and the Dakotas are indeed exporting many of their best-educated young, locating a headquarters in Butte, Billings, Bismarck, or the Black Hills, for example, could prove to be a demographic game-changer for an entire rural region, giving a youthful, tech-savvy, and highly dependable workforce a reason to plant roots close to home.

Rather than pick the winners of its corporate sweepstakes via quietly exclusionary or politically-biased criteria, Amazon might better live out its social justice-minded, equity-based creed by inviting applications from cities in America's Great Plains and Intermountain states, evaluating such places by what they have to offer—demonstrated work ethic, low rates of absenteeism and cost of living, affordable housing, underutilized infrastructure, high rates of civic participation and volunteerism, proximity to outdoor recreation and natural resources—rather than condemning them for their supposed lack of demographic fitness. And in return perhaps red and rural America might stop begrudging Amazon the energetic export and sale of its most cherished ideals.

In Praise of Barnyard English

A few years ago UNESCO sounded the alarm that half of the world's languages may become extinct by the end of our century. Serious hand-wringing and think-tank creating followed, along with a push by National Geographic, among others, to document and preserve the world's linguistic diversity under the rallying cry "Save a language. Save a culture." And yet nowhere in the necessary scramble to document the world's endangered indigenous tongues did I hear mention of what my farmer grandfather lovingly called Barnyard English.

If you grew up on or around a farm or ranch you know exactly the linguistic bumper crop to which I refer—that fecund, richly metaphoric language that seemed to roll off our grandparents' tongues but now seems awkward or incongruous on ours. My farm-girl grandmother Julia, for example, was fond of the phrase "pert near"—a contraction for "pretty near." Even now I can see her sitting at the kitchen table with a Coca-Cola in one hand and a grocery list in the other saying something like "That Mary Louise is pert near crazy" or "Your cousin Andrew pert near ran that little car of his into the ditch."

Pert near is a perfectly acceptable grammatical contraction, akin to substituting "I s'pose" for "I suppose." And yet how many rural kids turned circumspect urban professionals feel free to drop a "pert near" with a straight face and sans disclaimer in a boardroom, conference center, or lecture hall? Same goes for another favorite I came to love during the years I spent living in the rural South: the all-purpose verb "fixin'." Opening a meeting with "Next we're fixin' to hear our annual shareholder's report" strikes the average listener today as a mite shy of Ivy League.

The new school year that begins each autumn presents the perfect occasion for turning over a new linguistic leaf, returning, when the shoe fits, to the homespun phraseology of our ancestors. As it is we're often unduly sensitive about our perceived linguistic warts and especially thin-skinned when it comes to cultural pasts we've tried mightily as a people to transcend and evidently would prefer to forget. I remember, for example, the particular vehemence my elementary school teachers reserved for the word "ain't," which I was told was a word used by ignorant country people. To let an agrarian colloquialism like "pert near" back into our digital age vernacular in anything other than overproduced country music would seem erosive to most, a willful and egregious backsliding to the darker days when our livelihoods came hard hewn from the land not spiral-bound and collated at the office.

I, for one, am proud of the way my grandparents spoke. They came by their language via utility, necessity, and invention, rather than via the way most of their Gen X and Gen Y grandchildren came to speak "standard" English—by the more nefarious method long-preferred by assimilationists, hegemonists, imperialists, and cultural assassins—by decree, by fiat, by threat of public shaming for language that exits outside the urban norm and that carries still an objectionable whiff of the barnyard.

Of course to reintroduce the colorful Barnyard English our grandparents spoke so well to a digital generation would be a daunting task indeed. Charismatic young digerati are happy to indulge their elders with the occasional hokey utterance of "horse feathers!" but only with the same retro-ironical spirit that finds them buying up all the 1970s league bowling shirts at Goodwill with "Bob" stitched on the front pocket. Even the barnyard colloquialisms that once upon a time captured the urgency of youth itself—"sowing wild oats" or "making hay while the sun shines" have largely been put out to pasture.

I'm determined to stop censoring the agrarian English of my birthright for the sake of social expediency or professional convenience, and I want to empower my urban and rural students to do likewise. For those of us who were rural-raised to say that something is a "hard row to hoe" is language honed to a fine point—born of the experience of finding yourself knee-deep in the middle of a field surrounded by an impossible snarl of morning glory, pigweed, horseweed, or button weed. Similarly, to opine that "you can't dress up a pig" is a hard-won and wholly accurate truism that speaks equally to a pig's essential nature as well as to a pork-barrel politician's. And of course to say that one is really "goin' to town" is to recall a time in our populist gloaming when hitching up to travel to the nearest market village over impossibly muddy roads signified a difficulty requiring zealotry to overcome—a pluck and enthusiasm the feds have opaquely named "irrational exuberance."

One need only listen to the language of our current chief executives, bureaucrats, plutocrats, wonks, and academics to hear the utter absence of real agrarian wisdom. A farmer or rancher understands what it means when a politician misses his mark... is, in fact, so misguided in his or her aim that they couldn't hit the broad side of a barn. The yeoman likewise comprehends what it means when a hastily conceived idea or a lazy, good-for-nothin' policy is a dog that just won't hunt. To their credit the agrarian is less likely to cotton to today's unforgivable abstractions, those set down in phrases like "double down," "downsize," or, my personal favorite, "pivot."

Maybe I've missed the mark. Maybe the current generation of farmers' and ranchers' sons and daughters studying at colleges and universities now speak the language of the bureaucrat or CEO easily, breezily, and well. Still, I suspect even they recognize the utility, virility, energy, and integrity of the Barnyard English they've lost the courage or the cultural memory to speak. The other stuff, the scrap heap of buzzwords and Doublespeak and corporate euphemism, adds up to an agrarian linguistic nugget so apropos that it endures to this day as the perfect response for every professional evasion and obfuscation—*That's bullshit.*

Last Man Standing

Sometimes when I look out the window at this small farm I steward I realize I am shockingly alone. I've become a last man standing—last to bear my family name, the only son in a farm clan whose land has been in continuous ownership by my kin since 1855. It's a truer and sadder plot than ever I could have written, and one I never anticipated in a dreamy boyhood when my people seemed an abundant part of this place, inevitable as the dandelion, stalwart as the meadowlark.

Were the aloneness I feel simply personal, I wouldn't trouble you. But it's your loneliness, too, deep and black as topsoil, because as rural America goes, so go you. I could feed you the stats, but let's just call a spade a spade: the young don't stay, and if they do, it's straight to an apartment or condo in the city, leaving the countryside bereft of single twenty- and thirty-somethings.

Call me Chicken Little or Debbie Downer, but where among your many friends and neighbors and associates can you find, say, a young, single professional woman living in the countryside more than thirty miles from a major city? And what of the future viability of a place almost entirely devoid of young women? We've seen this movie before—Roanoke, the Wild West, the Yukon Territory, all starkly beautiful, perfectly unsustainable places.

Were I to write you a novel of a breadbasket place so fertile the world had never seen its equal, where corn yields 200 acres a bushel and stands in rows straight enough to please any minister, you might believe me. What if, turning the page, this miracle place of highest literacy and admirably fine schooling also turns out to be a place in whose hinterlands marriageable women are all but absent—like the land of the Amazons in Greek literature, only in reverse. The scenario thus written seems pure science fiction, and yet this fabulously precarious place exists. I know it because I live in it, and, if you are a rural American, so do you.

Bob Dylan famously sang you don't need a weatherman to know which way the wind blows, and you don't need a mathematician to dig the demographic equation: Brain drain + Lack of young rural singles = Death for the rural civilization whose survival is every bit as crucial to urban America as the hobbit's Shire was to the fate of Middle Earth.

I've lived my thirty-odd years on Planet Rural America deeply and dutifully studying its history and culture and, frankly, I'm fed up with the Pompeii of historical reenactments, "living history," and small-town fairs that ironically celebrate the very cultural mainstays that long ago passed away into ceremony (Railroad Days, Sauerkraut Days, Donna Reed Days) in much the same way that suburban housing developments are said to be named after the thing they destroy.

My family's seven generations of history here amid the tall corn has made of me an old man, and my habit of studying rural history in detail has made me dustier still. But the thing is, by rural standards, I'm young, and so are you, and there's something urban Americans can do to help their country cousins beyond visiting the farmers' market and paying state income taxes; they can acknowledge that folks living twenty or forty miles beyond the city lights ought to, by rights, have as good a chance at meeting an educated mate at the local convenience store or greasy spoon as an urban dude does chatting up a prospect at Starbucks. Entrepreneurial spirit has brought us country-dwellers the "wonders" of high-speed internet and digital cable, but I'd rather see an educated, dynamic, fiercely independent country girl stroll by my rural window than catch the latest "can't-miss" TV.

I could continue to stew here in the hills in prideful isolation (I will, and I do), but I'd be fiddling while Rome burned and the old generals expired or abandoned their posts. In the last decade alone I've lost my grandfather to cancer, and two too-young uncles to heart attacks. Their death and disappearance makes me free and bereft, blessed and cursed. I'm left to witness alone many farm mornings and evenings too beautiful to describe except in wish-you-were-here postcards. Still, I stay here, stand for here, because it's in my make-up, the way a horse lowers its head to stable as night comes.

But here's the thing: so long as we rural and small-town singles draw breath, voting with our feet for the sweetness that remains, there's a chance fate will find us where we live, and by our own mulishness and vestige of whatever it is that sustained our families here, deliver something like romance, something like manna.

We're Dying Here

Not so very long ago living a rural life was considered as near to healthful as a man or woman had the natural right to expect. At the turn of the twentieth century, in fact, selling life insurance to a rural citizen, especially if they were a farmer, made for good business. In that Populist gloaming plowmen and -women often outlived even the actuary's best estimates of their mortality, and no less than the *New York Times* reported that farmers were second only to clergymen in longevity, with forty out of every one hundred expected to live past seventy. And that was in 1893.

These days if you look closely at newspaper obituaries published in towns like mine across rural and small-town Middle America, you'll see a shocking number of fatalities of men and women in their forties, fifties, and sixties. Indeed, the week's crop of premature male deaths listed in our country newspaper includes two rural men ages 46 and 41 respectively. One, though our newspaper editor mercifully omits the fact, is widely understood to be a suicide.

Wrong-headed technocrats and cosmopolites would have us believe that such morbid numbers in morbidity—an average age of male death of just over forty-three years of age for our two weeks' worth of obituaries—represent local anomalies. But when homegrown anecdotal evidence joins with empirical research you have that rare beast otherwise known as fact—real, palpable and unspinnable.

The week my father's obituary ran in our local paper the average age of the male deceased barely topped the age of Social Security eligibility. My father, a farmer, passed away just a few months shy of his sixty-first birthday, and like any rural son I spent more time feeling guilty for whatever lifestyle and risk factors might have taken my dad from us too soon than engaged in the harder problem of solving for demographic x. I recalled my father saying, "You can't save people from themselves," and so I sat there, obit in hand, thinking that somehow his untimely passing must have been inevitable or somehow earned for failing to live up to some standard of how good and healthy people lived elsewhere—whoever and wherever they were. "No rest for the wicked and the good don't need it," my long-lived grandfather, likewise a farmer, always said, and for decades the plowman's corollary was that if you worked hard, stayed active, and "kept your nose clean and your breath sweet," as my Grampy was fond of saying, you would be a good bet to dance a jig at your 80th birthday.

Such sweet and enduring agrarian colloquialisms as these may have held true when Ike was president, but no longer. In today's rural America Baby Boomer sons who work the land are too often outlived by their own fathers, intimating a trend as spiritually and existentially heartbreaking as it is physiologically unthinkable.

Back when Barack Obama was the apple of rural America's eye I was invited to attend the President's Rural Economic Forum—more of an election-year PR opportunity for the White House, really, than a substantive discussion of rural issues. On my way out I picked up a publication no thicker than my small-town phonebook. *Jobs and Economic Security for Rural America* its title read, and like any Middle American swayed by the enticement of free literature, I flipped through what was intended to be the good news.

But as I thumbed to the middle of the government white paper—the burial place of choice for inconvenient truths—I learned that an urban resident was between 10 and 15 percentage points more likely to have attended college than a rural resident. A few more pages in a grim figure titled "Metropolitan and Non-metropolitan Mortality Rates," stopped me cold, showing as it did two sharply diverging lines. The graph was followed by this coy bit of GovernmentSpeak: "Since the early 1990s, mortality rates in urban and rural areas have diverged." The cause of the divergence was unclear, the report concluded in bureaucratese, but any rural family could have given the experts gathered that day an earful of examples of fifty-five- and sixty- and sixty-five-year-old nephews and uncles and fathers and even grandfathers taken too soon from them, and in the end would have reached the same sincere conclusion: "We're dying here."

Still graver, less sanitized stats can be confirmed in any number of reputable places, including a 2010 study in the *Journal of the American Medical Association* (JAMA), which found that three-quarters of the counties with the worst declines in life expectancy were rural. The authoritative JAMA study, reflecting changes in longevity between 1985 and 2010, returned a slew of rural counties where, for example, female life expectancies in places like Fayette County, Alabama, over the same twenty-five-year period had actually decreased by several years. Predictably the big losers were in a broad swath of non-metro counties in rural Middle American states such as Kentucky and Tennessee and Kansas and Oklahoma. On the flip side of the death coin was the big winner—New York City—with a net change of life expectancy over the same years of more than eight years for women and nearly thirteen for men.

The year my father passed away, for example, male life expectancy in the county where he was born and raised lagged behind that of the nearest state university city just a forty-minute drive away by nearly two and a half years.

The new national demographics show just as starkly the grim effects of geography on longevity, pinpointing and projecting where the aged are located—and it's decidedly not the frozen Heartland states one might have historically suspected—places like Minnesota, North Dakota, South Dakota, and Iowa that less than a decade ago ruled the roost of octogenarians. In the new math of morbidity states such as Iowa, Kansas, Nebraska, and the Dakotas barely topped single digits in percentage change from 2000 to 2010 in population aged eighty-five years and over, while states like Arizona, Colorado, and the rest of the West tripled and quadrupled their Midwestern counterparts, boasting a percentage change in number of octogenarians, nonagenarians, and centenarians living within their borders at close to 50 percent.

As politicians and planners initiate wishful campaigns designed to make their home states and regions the healthiest in America, one can't help but wonder if we once fiercely egalitarian rural Americans are okay accepting whole-hog the undemocratic notion that one's zip code can so dramatically determine one's attainment of a college education or longevity. The ruralites I knew as a boy would never have accepted a nearly fifteen-year longevity gap between New York, New York, and Floyd County, Kentucky, nor a nearly 45 percentage point difference in Bachelor's degree attainment between the residents of Iowa City, Iowa, and the denizens of the small rural towns caught in its outsized orbit. And since when did an aging rural-dweller, whether they are Nebraskan or Arkansan, face such a stark choice between living (and dying) where they love, and packing their bags to join the new winners in places with the highest percentage of folks aged 65 and over—places like Honolulu or Scottsdale or—surprise, surprise—Surprise City, AZ.

As recently as a generation ago America acknowledged the importance of offering its citizens, regardless of where they hung their hat, something close to geographic parity when it came to the essentials in life—clean air, decent water, passable schools, equitable access to basic health care and higher education—as part of the democratic ideal. No more. Now, indifferent or ignorant urbanites seem to regard rural living as a self-inflicted health hazard or risk factor—something akin to smoking or drinking or drug-addiction—in any case a dangerous lifestyle choice accompanied by grave consequences.

One day soon the well-preserved cosmopolite attending the wake of his country cousin will pause before his kinfolk's open casket and offer this dry-eyed if not sober lament: "If only the poor soul would have moved."

We Live and Die by Chemical Agriculture

On the 500-acre Century Farm of my boyhood an unspoken honor code applied: you applied your pesticides and your herbicides when the wind was calm, lest you evoke the sanction and shame of long-time neighbors. That honor code served as a compelling example of how community mores helped keep dangerous practices and environmental hazards in check better than any state regulator ever could.

Families, too, looked out for their own. "Go inside, kids, John's spraying," my mother or grandmother would say when John's red tractor pulled into the field south of our farmhouse towing the big boom sprayer. "Going inside" amounted to common-sense prevention for farm women and children in the face of dangerous chemicals suspected, even then, of being carcinogens.

John didn't notify us in advance when it was time to apply his pre- or post-emergent herbicides; he didn't need to. We knew he watched the extended forecast in order to choose the calmest day possible before he rolled his rig to a stop just beyond our shared fence-line. There he idled, adjusting the sprayer, quietly buying the adults time to get us inside. We understood implicitly that John would never intentionally harm us, that leaving the children of his farm neighbors choking in a toxic cloud would be as unthinkable as bathing his own babies in herbicides. To poison the children of the neighbors with whom you sat down to coffee would be a silly if not sinful thing to do.

Sadly, the common-sense Golden Rule honor code that held sway in the fields each spring in my 1980s boyhood no longer holds. And for those of us who still live on the farm but don't engage in chemical-intensive large-scale farming, the results are both toxic and terrifying. Farmers now routinely spray their seasonal herbicides in winds so fierce even private pilots think twice about taking off in them. We watch as wind-driven clouds of chemicals drift across our fields and into our children's lungs, onto our plants and trees, and, through the cracks and fissures of our old farmhouses, right into our very homes. Each spring the smell of lilacs mingles strangely with the reek of chemicals whose brand names we ruralites recognize on first whiff, the way a wine aficionado knows a particular vintage by nose.

These days, when I see the toxic cloud wafting toward me and mine I imagine the reaction many urban and suburban parents would have if they and their children were perennially soaked in chemicals. Indignant blogs would be posted, social media campaigns would be mounted, regulators would be called, heads would roll, and, sooner than later, the toxic practice would be dialed back or stopped altogether. These days even bombing raids come with advance warning to protect the lives of the innocent.

Of course, urban and suburban parents don't live here anymore. As the demographics clearly show they've mostly left our truly rural counties for a life in the bubble of our prosperous towns and cities, where children are better protected from chemical-intensive agriculture. Men like me who root down stubbornly in and near our native communities may be too headstrong, or else too expendable, to bother with moving. Often we fail to treat our own health with the reverence and sanctity with which we treat our children's or our animals'.

We rural dwellers live awash in chemicals; the number of human beings out here is dwarfed by the acres of chemical-ready, chemical-needy commodity crops. And the longevity statistics tell us the loss of life we suffer for our love of the open lands in which we live totals in the years, not in days or months.

Well-meaning and compassionate city-dwellers are often willing to open the gates of their feudal cities to the refugees of chemical-intensive agriculture, but even their magnanimity often comes with a shot of shame and judgment: "Aren't you glad you finally came to your senses and got out?" Those of us who stay on our acres know the "big sort" that finds the educated, higher-earning, and health-conscious living separate and unequal lives in our cities and suburbs isn't a long-term answer for a better, fairer, healthier, more equitable commonwealth.

Urban America spends far too much time vilifying its conventional farmers, so much so that many who practice this historically honorable profession carry with them a needless sense of guilt and complicity. That guilt and complicity sometimes turns into a compensatory, even retaliatory devil-may-care posture that sprays when it damn well pleases. It wrongly turns farmers into public outcasts, scapegoats, or pariahs, when in fact they are mostly good and grounded citizens.

Those of us whose respect for a rural heritage runs centuries deep wouldn't dream of asking our neighbors to stop spraying, though we might sometimes secretly wish it. We ask only that the common-sense honor code be reapplied. Our mutual love of the land means we who choose to live here are willing to retreat, to look the other way and "go inside" while you spray if only you'll do your part: choose wisely and raise your finger to the wind, if not for us then for our children.

The Rural Health Care Crisis Is Real

As lawmakers debate controversial health care bills in Washington they should bear in mind a recent report by the CDC showing life expectancy declining for rural Americans. Ruralites, the Center concludes, are more likely to die from the top five causes of death than fellow citizens living in cities and suburbs.

The report mentions a litany of potential reasons for the alarming inequity, including poorer access to high-quality hospital care and doctoring, and lifestyle factors such as smoking, obesity, and physical inactivity. While it took the CDC until 2017 to publish these findings, the government has known about the disparity since at least 2011, when similarly disquieting information was quietly distributed to those of us invited to attend Barack Obama's Rural Economic Forum.

The latest study published in *JAMA Internal Medicine* delivers still more morbid news to those living in rural counties not otherwise considered destinations. As Joel Auchenbach reports in his May 8 article in the *Washington Post*, "A baby born in Summit County, Colorado, has a life expectancy of nearly 87 years, but in some counties the life expectancy is more than 20 years lower."

While the latest *JAMA* study requires a subscription to access, the 2014 longevity data kept by healthdata.org does not. There an interactive map shows more of the same: longevity at nearly eighty-seven years for Summit County, Colorado—a full ten years above life expectancy in some of the less populated, poorer, more rural counties in the southeast corner of that state. The longevity gap between Oglala Lakota County in South Dakota and Summit County totals a heartbreaking twenty years.

In long-lived Iowa a child born today is likely to live a relatively long life when compared to other states, still the discrepancy in longevity between rural and urban mimics national trends. Comparing Marshall County (average life expectancy 77.3 years) with Johnson County (82.08) reveals a nearly five-year life expectancy gap for a child born today in counties whose county seats are separated by less than ninety miles as the crow flies.

As a seventh-generation rural citizen who chooses to live on a farm I find the CDC's conclusions both self-evident and heartbreaking. Those of us who make our home far from easily accessible outdoor recreation, hospitals, and specialized clinics have woken up to the grave health disadvantages we face. Granted, we may be more doctor-adverse by age or ideology, and yet the doctors who might treat our maladies are often a thirty- or forty-mile drive away—double that if what we suffer is a mental illness, a psychological disorder, or some other chronic condition requiring a specialist.

The debate over longevity-endowed America's moral responsibility to its country cousins is an urgent one. And the disparity we feel is not just in health care but in infrastructure, legal services, law enforcement, social services, education, and more. As tax dollars shift to places called "smart cities" and "knowledge hubs" (university and research hospital cities, and affluent suburbs, exurbs, and resort communities) rural Americans in places like Iowa find ourselves largely bereft of the services we need (and characteristically don't expect) to lead healthful, equitable lives.

Rural America is strong of mind and doesn't need high-minded paternalism from society's more affluent and healthy "winners." What we need is an acknowledgement that our health, welfare, and well-being matter to a nation whose rural citizens are now a conspicuous and little-covered demographic minority (just 15 percent of the U.S. population and falling, according to the *Washington Post* article cited above.) Now more than ever caring urbanites and suburbanites living in places where MLK's "Injustice anywhere is a threat to justice everywhere" is taken as creed must heed the health care injustice plaguing Middle America. And we rural Americans need to help our legislators understand that King's "anywhere" is here and now.

The Gift of Homecoming

Each and every fall fresh-faced men and women make their way to the fifty-yard line to await with bated breath the results of their classmates' vote for homecoming king and queen. Hours later, after the last of the pigskins and fleecy blankets have been put to rest, they wait in anticipation for the moment when their newly elected king and queen will lead them out onto the gymnasium floor for the night's first dance. Time slows to an agreeable standstill.

Homecoming is a concept an agrarian like me can get behind, whole-hog and wholesale. It's not yet tarnished by the sexual excesses and psycho-dramas of prom, with its perennial assault on the virginal and its too-steep psycho-social toll on the unpopular and undesirable. Homecoming shares not just a season but a spirit with Thanksgiving, that most irreproachable of agrarian holidays in which we still somehow insist on trading blessings and homemade casseroles in lieu of Chinese-made baubles.

At root homecoming is a collegiate conceit, and as such it cannot help but perpetuate inequities of privilege, class, and upward social mobility. The earliest of U.S. homecomings, hosted at such venerable institutions as the University of Missouri, were thoroughly steeped in the notion of symbolic pedigree, cultivating a tradition whereby the alma mater, Latin for nourishing mother, would welcome her most successful graduates back to hearth and home.

The return of native sons and daughters, these captains of industry, these movers and shakers of State Street and Wall Street, to their college "home" functioned as a ritual reminder of wholesome parentage and all due filial loyalty. In one carefully planned weekend homecoming spirits would be lifted, purse strings would be loosened, and pocketbooks would be opened wide in honor of the ivy walls and ivy towers that had birthed lucrative careers and lush lives. And still today the University of Missouri model is alive and well; homecoming, for proud alumnae who "done good," is an event not to be missed, occupying a privileged spot in the professional's autumnal calendar alongside such seasonal save-the-dates as quarterly business meetings and getaway vacations.

Still, one cannot help but entertain the countless ways left-behind communities might be transformed if and when the cognoscenti who many moons ago left for greener professional pastures in college towns and metropolitan areas regarded their hometowns with the depth of loyalty and material support they yearly bestow on their football-endowed alma maters. What if each and every autumn generations of the good and caring people fostered in our homespun hometowns and home places returned to their childhood haunts by the tens of thousands from the places they've made their handsome livings as adults? More importantly for our struggling villages and neighborhoods, many of which are a single failed bond issue or sewer upgrade away from total disincorporation, what if these prosperous homecomers brought not just their good cheer, good looks, and good health, but also their good credit?

Many of these high-flyers make invaluable contributions to their colleges and universities when they return for homecoming. In 2013 the Lily School of Philanthropy at Indiana University relayed the annual numbers calculated by the USA Giving Foundation. Charitable giving to education, they reported, had increased a whopping 7 percent from 2011 to 2012, despite deep recession, to an annual total of $41.3 billion. Of this, approximately $31 billion had gone to four-year colleges and universities. Collectively, these well-endowed boosters of college and university alma maters have the wherewithal to positively alter their hometowns' destiny forever. According to the League of Cities and the U.S. Census the number of municipalities in America totals roughly twenty thousand.

What if the $31 billion in charity given to college and universities alone in the calendar year 2011–12 was instead given to the small towns who nurtured these same big donors for the first eighteen years of their lives? The result would be approximately $1.5 million per annum per municipality in charitable giving to the sorts of forgotten places where many Baby Boomers cut their teeth. That's $1.5 million per town for sewer upgrades, libraries, firehouses, playgrounds and playhouses, small-town parks and community centers.

It would be Christmas in October.

Of course moral and monetary support is a two-way street. Most homecomers to small towns aren't feted with hall-of-fame inductions, honorary degrees, ribbon-cuttings, and building dedications as they are at the colleges and universities where they happily matriculated and where they willingly return each and every fall. Perhaps part of the blame lies with the towns that have yet to roll out the red carpet for their AWOL sons and daughters—yet to unambiguously celebrate their cash crop of human resources, even if that crop long ago uprooted and took itself to market elsewhere. For some of our hard-pressed towns and neighborhoods how to host a can't-miss "homecoming" might just be a thirty-one-billion-dollar question.

In the end America's more fortunate sons and daughters have money enough to lay laurel wreaths and silver dollars at the feet of both their alma maters—hometown and home university—and yet the latter of these nourishing mothers receives almost all their financial support, while the former receives, at best, token moral support. Surely the highest-flying of highest achievers feel, or ought to feel, a fierce appreciation for the life-sustaining succor of both campus and home community.

Granted, one comes with the allure of winning football and a backdrop of youthful coeds, Grecian columns, and white-hot stadium lights, while the other may be a struggling town or economically depressed neighborhood more difficult to cheerlead in practice. Still, both college and home community have a legitimate claim as seed beds and nurseries for valuable human resource crops destined to bloom elsewhere. If our rural- and inner-city-born professionals are not yet in a position to vote with their heart, or their feet, for the home places that fed and clothed them since they were in diapers, they might at least consider voting for them with their dollars.

Rural Ghouls

Contrary to its rural roots the All Hallows of my lifetime has always been something of a town holiday, and little wonder. Trick-or-treating at the end of a long country lane is next to impossible, and farming can be macabre enough as it is. The sight of missing digits and severed arms are real here where I hang my hat and sharpen my plowshare, and especially so around harvest time.

Ask any farmer whether he relishes schlepping the kiddos into town and idling in the car while they go a-begging for Grade-A goodies from commuter moms and dads snug in their bedroom communities, and if he's in a truth-telling mood, he'll tell you otherwise. Seeing his kids dressed up to please and placate the folks with the best candy and the best jobs is a bit too near to real life to strike him as harmless allegory.

When urban America needs a really good scare it typically turns to the countryside it privately fears and long ago left for dead—the place where the rest of us choose to make our homes and raise our families despite long odds. How could it be otherwise? City folks have come calling here for generations when the harvest moon rises in the sky, looking to get back in touch with the psycho-active aspects of lives they've sanitized for the sake of safety and a good clean living made in office park or skyrise.

It's the NIMBY phenomenon all over again, only this time in a beguiling guise, and it's the latest in drive-bys—a quick trip to the hinterlands to pick a plump pumpkin, a boon Saturday afternoon for the kiddos at the corn maze or the petting zoo, a heart-pounding Friday night at some decrepit fallen-down house someone's grandparents actually lived in. It's tragically ironic: the house of horrors they're white-knuckling in likely fell to its current state of ruination in the 1970s or 1980s when there were no young people willing to live in it when they could instead be living high on the hog in the nearest metro or university town.

The young citified couple in their skinny jeans will gladly pay their ten bucks to enter the haunted house where local high school kids will leap out at them wielding the axes and chainsaws they probably brought from home and actually know how to use. It's a great date night, sure, a relatively cheap thrill, to go whistling through the graveyard of your country cousins once a year, then return home to laugh it off over a pumpkin latte.

Don't mistake me for the Grinch Who Stole All Hallows. My rural family has hosted its share of frighteningly good haunted houses over the more than one hundred and sixty years we've haunted our own Heritage Farm. But when we donned the Frankenstein masks we were performing for our rural family, friends, and neighbors using the clothes and hats and handkerchiefs we actually put to frequent use the other three hundred and sixty-four days of the year. We were straight-up repurposing, not nudge-nudge, wink-wink cultural reappropriating.

Contrast our homegrown haunts with the reality of contemporary Halloween in the suburbs, where for a single week in late October it's as rare as a Willy Wonka's golden ticket, which is to say as rare as hen's teeth, to find a pair of pinstripe "farmer" overalls on the racks at the local Goodwill or Salvation Army. Ditto the straw hat and handkerchief and work boots that practically scream farmer in the eyes of a screen generation. Of course, before these threads became the Fright Night clothes of choice, they belonged to the farmer, who dressed his scarecrow in his duds so the crows might mistake the dressed-up staves of the cross for the spooking arms of the farmer himself. That's costumery with an appropriately utilitarian and rural twist.

Urbanists would have you believe that their perennially elaborate (and expensive) game of dress-up is a harmless enough homage to their country cousins. Their great-grandfather was a farmer, they'll insist, intimating that his willingness to work the land somehow confers on them the ability to spoof his stock and trade.

Or consider the much maligned, much snickered-at-in-urban-circles farmer's daughter. Most of the paper-pushers at the office Halloween party would, after a cocktail or two, shudder at the thought of pulling their real-life daughter from her $80 million suburban schoolhouse and enroll her in an under-resourced rural school, to say nothing of giving her a dignified role to play in the running of an actual commodity crop farm they've purchased to work themselves. But they wouldn't think twice of dolling themselves up as the naughty-but-nice cultural icon they've played a large part in turning into a disgraced and defamed sex symbol—a laughable cardboard cut-out light on realism and heavy on cleavage.

And isn't that always the way? We wear the clothes of the people we've successfully subjugated or undermined or simply cheated to the point of decimation. Not too many Victorian Americans could be found clamoring for Indian feathers and headdresses until Sitting Bull and Geronimo were roundly defeated and widely paraded around the world's fairs and Wild West shows. Once these formerly fearsome warriors and national bugaboos were subdued and safely under armed guard, however, Americans practically tripped over themselves to dress the part of the Indian warrior.

Or consider the early Jazz Age fashion sensation popular among urban gals keen to dress the part of the farmerette at exactly the moment in history when they had left the farm in droves to work as secretaries and stenographers in the city. Need more proof of how we carry on once we've removed the existential threat of the Other? Type "Farmer's Daughter Costume" into the search engine of your favorite online retailer and you'll see something that looks XXX—and I'm not referring to triple extra-large. Can you think of any other icon of American virtue and ingenuity so thoroughly caricatured and crassly sexualized?

Or you could spend the ghastly holiday in a horror movie marathon, where you could get your scream on with the original 1984 Stephen King version of *Children of the Corn,* or the 2009 made-for-TV remake filmed in the swampy bottomlands just a half mile from my farm, and on the town square in my childhood county seat. Or try on a newer version of the rural slasher flick such as 2011's *Husk.* If those rural scares fail to titillate, you could always go old-school with *Deliverance,* a film that gave new meaning to the term "squeal like a pig" and scared a generation of young men and women both from banjos and from making a home in the boonies.

It's the same old story, really. Urban America wants a yearly dose of the horrors it otherwise congratulates itself on leaving behind—depravity and poverty, social isolation and eerie silences, chainsaws and farm implements gone awry.

Look more closely, however, and you see a real-life ax-murder playing out in America's empty acres—the whodunit of the millions of farmers and their families forced from their livelihoods in the last forty years, or the 70 percent of North American farmland soon to be awaiting an unironic heir willing to wield sharp instruments in the frighteningly difficult task of wresting a living from the land.

If I had one wish this coming Halloween season, it would be that rural America quit being so complicit in aping its own proud heritage for the amusement of folks whose Disneyfied image of the countryside comes from the once-a-year hayrack rides and corn mazes we ruralites all too willingly stage for their giddy delight. Sure, humoring city slickers may be good for business or agri-tourism, but it's a dagger to the heart and soul of the places we live, and increasingly, die.

Cyber Monday in the Country

To hear the newspapers and magazines tell it, Black Friday is so 2012—the year when its grandeur and its share of the market seemed to peak. Ever since, pundits claim, we have been falling out of love with this caveman holiday in favor of a newer, niftier flame: Cyber Monday.

The respective names of these kissin' cousin commercial holidays say it all: one darkly ominous—black comedy writ large—the other clean, white, and highly palatable. The rise of Cyber Monday neatly parallels the tastes of wealthier, better-connected North Americans currently fueling the growth in seasonal e-commerce. In 2016 *Fortune* magazine gleefully predicted that more Americans would shop online than go to stores over the four-day holiday weekend. And yet, cool or uncool, Black Friday is disproportionality important to the bottom-line of many rural and small-town citizens lacking ready access to online deals.

Commerce-shaming, not unlike the weight-shaming and body-shaming many cosmopolites decry, is now the order of the day, with multiple news outlets arguing that Cyber Monday is the morally superior alternative to its cruder caveman cousin. "Here's Why You Shouldn't Go to the Store on Black Friday," reads a C-Net headline, listing reasons ranging from the limbic/lizard brain (the visceral fear-mongering implicit in mentions of Black Friday fights, tramplings, and mobs) to the highly rational and intellectual (the smart shopper gets better deals on Cyber Monday). Meanwhile, sporting goods retailing giant REI now closes its doors on both Thanksgiving and Black Friday, winning praise from socially-conscious, internet-endowed consumers while effectively shutting out those without adequate online access.

Such high-minded reasons for avoiding Black Friday may make perfect sense for metropolitans snugged up with their high-speed broadband and distrust of the *demos* in democracy. But in the nation's rural and small-town places Black Friday is not yet a cultural villain. And we dodo birds who still indulge such commercial dinosaurs as 6 a.m. doorbuster deals are not the willfully backslid, backward, morally bankrupt plebes we're often written up to be.

According to the FCC's Broadband Progress Report, 39 percent of rural Americans (23 million people) lack access to broadband. By contrast only 4 percent of urban Americans lack access to the same. Sophisticated Cyber Monday shoppers who look down their noses at the pigs in a chute who line up for Black Friday in-store deals may want to recall the frustrations they felt with digital commerce back in, say, 2007, when their broadband speeds likely approximated those achieved by many and small-town rural Americans today...on a good day.

If Thanksgiving means sharing the great American melting pot with those who do not share your racial profile, education level, ZIP code, earning potential, and technological literacy, then the fully analog experience of Black Friday is as down-to-earth and grassroots patriotic as it gets. Those who disdain Black Friday would do well to remember that buying and selling are social rather than solitary acts, begging the question: whose actions are more societally valuable—the communal shopper waiting their turn with the Walmart throngs, or the digital shopper high in their cool silicon-blue tower interacting with no one save Google.

While arguably not as environmentally friendly as the UPS and Fed-Ex-driven Cyber Monday, the miles we Black Fridays drive to our nearest big-box stores stimulate a much wider cross-section of the economy—from oil and gas to food and entertainment. For us Black Friday is an immersive, egalitarian, all-day experience—a modern folkway—not a mere commercial interruption in an afternoon of smooth chardonnay, soft slippers, and "clean" e-commerce.

Part III:

Holidays

Holidays on Ice

Like many adult ruralites I've suffered my share of holiday guilt and grief—much of it self-imposed, and the rest imposed by others who feel I ought to celebrate after their fashion: big sweaters, loads of hot dishes, a surfeit of idle chit-chat with distant relatives who return to our country towns and ancestral farms just long enough to collect their gift cards. In many ways the traditional holiday fete piques the rural stoic archetype. Don't get me wrong: my beef isn't with the sacred spirit of the season, but with the straightjacket many of us feel compelled to put on in order to celebrate it.

Family holiday fetes can be downright claustrophobic for free-range men and women. My Uncle Wayne, a self-professed hillbilly engineer and farm-owner from Pikeville, Kentucky, used to grab me at those inevitably claustrophobic moments during family Christmas on the farm and say, "Hey, fella, come outside and let's smoke a joint." Uncle Wayne's joint was actually a Swisher Sweet cigar, but our mission was the same: get out of the house for some much needed air and a fresh perspective. Needless to say, Uncle Wayne had married into the family.

Second, the holidays' requisite uniforms can't help but confine. My family members, mostly farmers or laborers of various stripes, typically wore work clothes for their workaday lives. The duds they donned the other three hundred and sixty-four days a year weren't especially shabby or smelly—they didn't reek like a deep fat fryer or an open grease pit or a pig pen—they just looked comfortably worked in. For men and women who worked outside most of their lives, holiday events seemed to require donning the clothes of the office worker—a collared shirt or "nice" sweater, some trousers with a pleat in them, gratuitously thick socks and fuzzy slippers that conferred an anomalous softness on their wearers. Seeing my grandfather—an Osh Kosh B'gosh overalls grain farmer and seed corn salesman—dressed in some obligingly fleecy Christmassy flannel made him seem suddenly foreign to me, as I am sure he was to himself. And maybe it's because he seemed uncomfortable in his own skin on Xmas that I began to think that everyone around me might have felt a little compelled to put on an act. For whose benefit I was never certain, and I'm still not.

Finally, there's the holiday celebration protocol itself. Is there an opt-out? A none-of-the-above? Is the son or daughter of rural America allowed to say, a la the Herman Melville character Bartleby, that they prefer not to show up at 10 a.m. on Christmas Day freshly showered and already clawing at that uncomfortable turtleneck he desperately wants out of? Is a grown man or woman permitted to say they'd rather spend all or part of the special day in their workshop, or catching up on their newspaper reading, or studying their new *How to Speak Italian* book? Maybe, but there will surely be hell to pay. The holiday mafia will see to it that our escapist tendencies are sunk. After all, they know where we live.

These days I feel this most sacred of seasons ought not to make people feel uncomfortable in their own skin, or create an overwhelming need to meet the expectations of others. If the rural stoic is really and truly a loner, let him be alone if he chooses. If she's an inveterate traveler, let her experience Christmas in Rome one year and New Year's in Key West the next. If he's a homebody who wants nothing more than to eat auntie's cookies and open up gifts carefully packed with return receipts, let him have his commercial holiday without undue guilt or criticism.

In other words let the overlarge and undersized shirts and sweaters pulled out of gift-wrapped boxes each holiday season serve to remind us of an important chestnut: the way we celebrate the holidays need not be one-size-fits-all.

Christmas Wishes

Sadly, in-store layaway and the glossy holiday catalogues known as Wish Books now belong to the days when slow-moving dinosaurs like Sears and Montgomery Ward roamed the big-box plains in the salad days before the credit card meteor hit and changed everything. Both were fixtures in a rural childhood, and a regular life-saver for cash-poor parents like mine determined to beat the Christmas rush. While layaway once had cachet, it's now mostly relegated to discount stores where it's known by slick euphemisms. After all who wants to "layaway" when you can "reserve," "hold," or "select"?

Not so many moons ago, before in-store charge cards, a proud citizen could march up to the layaway counter with their head held high. Typically the layaway department was tucked away in the back next to the fitting rooms and managerial offices, far from the madding crowds. There a hushed civility predominated. Whereas the back room in a guy-only joint invariably turned into a den of depravity, the back room in the department stores of my youth felt something like an elderly woman's closet—regal without being uppity. Layaway clerk was a plum job—like being postmaster in a town of one hundred. You could expect a stampede between Thanksgiving and Christmas, but for most of the rest of the year your dance card stayed blissfully empty.

The dignified ladies who ran layaway presided over an impressively diverse intermingling of race, class, and ethnicity. In their department blue-collar Sally Fields types like my mom mingled with the pillbox and gloved specimens of earlier generations, for whom layaway was an emblem of financial discretion and a point of pride. Both classes of women knew what they wanted, how much it would cost, how long it would take to get, and how sweet it would be when, at last, the object of their delayed gratification became theirs.

All that came to an end when the world's largest retailer, Walmart, announced it would no longer accept layaways, arguing that the option discouraged their customers from signing up for the Walmart card. Hardly anyone noticed the proposed phase-out, though petitiononline.com did post a petition stating, in part, "For families, Walmart's layaway plan means satisfaction at Christmas, birthdays, and other gift-giving holidays & birthdays. There are a lot more people out there that, without layaway, will not be able to afford buying Christmas presents at Walmart."

In announcing the phase-out the press release cited declining demand, online shopping, gift cards, and no-cost credit alternatives as reasons for the stoppage. For the few who cared the executive vice president of store operations for the Walmart stores division offered "one last opportunity to use layaway service this Christmas season." Layaway was a system tailor-made for straight-up hard-working folks and the eager kids who hoped to become the proud owners of whatever hard-won gifts awaited them behind the counter. It taught us that what was worth having was worth waiting for, and along with the venerable Sears

Wish Book, served as a bright star in our wintertime commercial constellation.

When the Wish Book arrived in our rural route mailbox my sister and I would ring in the season with a game we called Playing Pages. To begin we had only to declare whether we claimed the left or right pages. Whatever was on our side of the Wish Book as we flipped through the glossy holiday annual become ours, at least in our overactive imaginations. Thus it happened that a boy of ten or twelve could acquire such manly things as a new electric razor, and an adolescent girl could count a satin negligee among her daily finds. Sometimes the boy ended up with the negligee and that was fun and enlightening, too.

The Wish Book served as our own country advent, counting down the days while determining the limits of gifting possibility each holiday season, defining and describing the forms our desires could take, like the Wells Fargo mail-order catalogues of old. Playing Pages was simply to let the eye acquire the object of its desire, to pour over every detail until we had the image committed to our covetous memories. With visual aids like these who needed sugar plum fairies? In school and on Main Street the country women in our lives taught us that it was impolite to stare, but in the world of the Wish Book staring became coin of the realm. When my sister and I made our Christmas lists we negotiated between the rational and the irrational, the possible and the impossible.

Not surprisingly, in days when layaway is now passé, gift-cards have become the gift-giving norm and "wish lists" have turned into laundry lists dutifully filled by bleary-eyed parent-shoppers, such wintertime accoutrements of a rural childhood find themselves in steep decline. In recent years Sears quietly issued a press release announcing that it had moved its venerable Wish Book online, citing better access there for anxiety-ridden parents. "Now instead of running from store to store searching for the most popular toys of the seasons," the press release quotes the president of Sears Direct as saying, "customers can find what they need by shopping online at wishbook.com." While the release hastened to add that the print copy would still be available for purchase at approximately half the cost of a novel newly released in paperback, the catalog's free delivery days were history.

In issuing their respective decrees announcing the new holiday normal the corporate elves at Walmart and Sears forgot that the Wish Book and layaway were never merely for holiday-stressed professional parents who, as the announcement put it, "anxiously brace for the worst." After all, while parents may have earnestly wanted a convenient worry-free holiday season, we country kids were all too happy to indulge in the season's definitive act: the lost art of good-spirited wishing, and the delayed gratification that made such powerful yearning possible.

May Day

The First of May, as our grandparents knew, begs a holiday. Easter lay weeks in the past. April Fools is a blip, a gimmick—a bad joke or a left-handed prank. Memorial Day, meanwhile, waits weeks away, beckoning with a three-day weekend if you work in the city, but promising only more time in the field if your kin farm, as do mine.

Farm kids both, my folks first initiated us early to the mysterious rites of May, when the crops first send their green shoot up through the earth—a little vegetable maypole—and the green haze of next month's fodder gradually overspreads the hillsides. For country kids like us it was usually our first time outside in a light jacket, or, if we were lucky, in long sleeves, and we were feeling our oats.

Back then May Day proved tailor-made for the historical moment—an epoch when an enterprising parent could take two or three or four rambunctious munchkins, give them a stack of waxy Dixie Cups with a nice floral print, a bunch of bagged candy, and some homemade popcorn or peanuts to shell, and create for them a "learning experience." A paper-punch and a pipe cleaner later you had a makeshift basket and a handle you could hold May by—passing its prodigality on for the sharing.

But the best part of May Day wasn't stuffing our baskets—though playing springtime Santa for a day went straight to our kid heads—it was the hocus-pocus disappearing act awaiting us just the other side of the doorbells we rang. Into the car we scrambled with a cardboard flat full of overflowing Dixie Cups, making Mom slow down for the tight curves on the road into town for fear our cups would runneth over. Like Santa, we made our list, populated it with the both naughty and nice, and headed off to town, where our aunts and most of our schools friends waited: sitting city ducks.

When we arrived, Mom's ancient Olds idling in someone else's drive, one of us little imps, crouching low like a solider, would race around the car, scamper to the door, ring the doorbell, and beat it the heck back to the backseat, the car already rolling when we slammed the door shut. Then we kids would rubberneck around to watch our half-suspecting victims open the door and blink into the sun like Punxsutawney Phil on the second of February before reaching down for the little grail we'd filled. It was like fair-weather trick-or-treating only better and without any of the "Oh my, how scary you children look!" play-acting. Who wanted to perform like a circus monkey for an adult when you could have it your way, ring the doorbell, disappear like Invisible Man, then stick around to watch the gray-hairs scratch their salt and pepper at your miraculous front-door offering.

For all that delicious joy, however, we don't celebrate May Day much anymore. Today most kids only see a Maypole on American Movie Classics or when they're dragged along by their parents to a Renaissance fair where May Day lives in the past along with knights and ladies, warriors and wenches. The First of May now slips by with nary a dance, distressed damsel, or Dixie Cup.

When we miss marking May, we miss much. We let corporate America set our seasonal clocks—first to Valentine's Day, then Easter, then Memorial Day, with only a brief interlude for last-minute shopping in between. We conveniently forget the old agrarian calendar when May 1 was as good a reason to join hands with your neighbors around the Maypole as it was to hope your ribbon would get tied up with your sweetheart's and you'd have to figure out how to untangle yourselves. Elders looking on, you'd be left to determine where you began and where your sweetie left off—just like real life. Somehow love as a colorful mess of ribbons—an impossible knot you and your partner had to figure out how to undo and redo to fully appreciate its strength—died along with our observance of May.

The country families of my youth valued May Day in their bones. They knew it as an overspreading warmth that had them ready, when the grass greened, to tap their toes and engage in a little good-natured mischief. Today's generation of children, most of whom will never take up the plow or negotiate foaling season as a rite of spring, would do well to keep the tradition alive. We can help them by taking the time to fill their baskets to brimming. And when they look at us, puzzled at this seemingly inexplicable spring holiday, we can tell them, the old mischief dancing in our eyes: think of it as Thanksgiving in May.

Mothers' Day

I remember feeling awkward as a child when prodded by my parents to mumble to my gran, "Happy Mother's Day." Back then I felt grandmas and moms were as different as Coke and Pepsi, Apple and IBM, or Sonny and Cher. You didn't dare confuse the two, and if you did, woe unto you.

Grandmothers, I foolishly thought, had graduated from motherhood. They were decorated veterans of a good and just war they no longer needed to fight. They had retired after countless years of faithful service, earned the rank of professor emeriti, Motherhood Studies.

When Mother's Day arrives each May, I realize just how wrong I was—how much the yeoman's work of grandmothering deserves equal praise and decoration, especially for those of us raised or co-raised by grandmothers with the passion, dedication, creativity, cultivation, and vision the best moms bring. It's a time ripe for putting the plural back in Mothers' Day.

For most of my childhood my mom left the house early in the morning to work at flower and gift shops. This was not the June Cleaver motherhood she had imagined; it was working motherhood by necessity. Still, it left my sister and me with an unexpected boon: the power of a co-mother of force, fun, and magnitude.

In fact, Gran co-mothered a whole generation of us—the children of working parents needing to make a living. She might simply have retired the badge of motherhood, hung it up to play bridge or pinochle in her retirement years. She might have claimed as her just reward for years of service a well-deserved relocation to West Palm Beach or Santa Barbara. Everyone would have understood had she, after raising four children of her own on the farm, grandmothered by correspondence and by greeting card.

Instead she took us all in, feed us, perplexed us, inspired us, and compelled us. While our parents worked to keep the lights on, Gran labored to remind us that there was something more to life than working, that getting older didn't necessarily have to mean having less fun. While my parents spent much of their energy protecting me (from rough-and-tumble older cousins, from the ever-present dangers of TV, from the supposed evils of too much sugar…the list goes on) Gran mothered us into a world of full-on go-forth engagement.

At my grandmother's funeral, my cousin Rodney recalled one of his favorite stories of our co-mother. My parents had left for their respective jobs that morning with a firm admonition to Gran that she not, under any circumstances, allow me to play tackle football with my older cousins—something I wanted with my whole heart to do. Rodney recalled how Gran waited until she heard the door click to turn to me and say, "Now go out there and play!"

In my book and in many others grans are not mother's helpers, mothers-once-removed, or mother's assistants: they're mothers of distinction. Mother's Day is a grand time to thank a grandmother (or aunt)—without the least bit of sheepishness or self-consciousness—for her years of voluntary and often thankless service.

In that way, and in so many others, she's not just a mother of distinction. She's a mother by definition.

Our Ancestors Sleep Down the Road

In the nation's Heartland we're neighborly with the dead most days, not just on days when we're told.

As a general rule cemeteries powerfully occupy the Urban Mind just once per year, on Memorial Day, as calendar and commerce dictate. For my seventh-generation farm family, however, the graveyard amounts to a kind of annex, a neighborhood living room. In the small meadow beside the Civil War-era gravestones we have wept and picnicked as well as cursed and laughed, finding sadness and solace there not for one day, but for many days. At various times my cousins held the prized contract to keep our pioneer cemetery, circa 1842, mowed. Trimming around our ancestors' tombstones earned my cousins some extra income, and it also brought them face to face with their long-gone kin, as well as to their knees in a posture ideal for both weeding and penitence.

My farm grandfather and father, meanwhile, worked here for free—cutting back brush in the dog days of July and otherwise grooming the place within an inch of its life. As a teenager I could sometimes be convinced to join them, rubbing sleep from my eyes as I chiseled an ever larger chip on my shoulder, thinking about how unfair it was that we donated our labor for free, risking life and limb with balky chainsaws for a cemetery where fully half of the graves had been abandoned a half-century before I took my first breath. At the time it seemed a shameful waste—evidence of my family's predilection for devoting its time and treasure to lost causes and sinking ships—fatalism almost by definition.

Now I see things differently. I see our local boneyard as a rural "third place"—Ray Oldenburg's term for the necessary, free-admission spaces in our lives that lie beyond work and home. The pioneer cemetery functions for us as a house of memory. I remember burying my grandfather here just two days before my 29th birthday, and laying my uncle to rest after a sudden heart attack took him in middle age. I recall planting my grandmother in her chosen spot beneath the good Midwestern loam as I listened to my father's own forebodings of death, our mutual sweat and tears mingling in the dirt. If I didn't see to it that he was planted here beside his mother and father in a simple pine box he would personally haunt me, he pledged. And he meant it.

Two short years later I spent whole afternoons filling the holes I'd made sinking his heavy limestone memorial deep into the ground. I recall my second cousin Joel, trustee to this small collection of Union and farm dead, arriving unexpectedly one afternoon to help. Shovel in hand, he implored me not to feel as if I had to plant my roots here, not to get myself "locked into" the family pattern my father had, following familial obligation to the grave.

Still, to lay one's head and one's hat a quarter mile down the road from where your ancestors sleep each night is a point of pride. To put one's world right requires that one dream the dream of the living and the dead in some simultaneity, walking between them—life and death—as between two friends down a twilit gravel road.

Father's Day and the Film That Gets Rural America Right

Every quarter century or so moviemakers remember that rural America exists and decide to film this or that blockbuster in the nation's back yard. Hollywood perennially misunderstands and mischaracterizes Middle America and its people, so it's no big reveal that so many hinterland epics have pulled the bait and switch—flattering us with their attentions before caricaturing us all the way to the box office.

Bridges of Madison County and *A Thousand Acres* come to mind unless you're of a mind to consider adultery, abuse, dread diseases, poisoning, madness, jealousy, and treachery quintessentially rural traits, and good luck to you if you do. Against such sensationalist precedents as these *Field of Dreams* offers a bright contrast. It's fair to say the film gets us right, or at least as near to right as any big-budget flick shot in rural America about rural America.

In the thirty years since "If you build it he will come" became a cultural mantra everywhere dreams are grown, Midwesterners who were still greenhorns back in 1989 have grown up alongside the iconic motion picture that's matured along with us—the one to which we answer no matter how far we roam. Now, hoeing the long row into middle age, we've come, many of us have, to a deeper appreciation of what made *Field of Dreams* ring so true to the rural American experience when first it graced our movie screens more than thirty years ago.

Contrary to their public image, farmers like Ray Kinsella have big imaginations. Folks living on the coasts like to think of the nation's food producers as stoical, by-the-book, don't-rock-the-boat types, but anyone who grew up on a farm or ranch or who works on one now will tell you farmers and ranchers are more like Kinsella in their visionary drive than the passionless, by-the-numbers businessmen, actuaries, or accountants they're often typecast as. Indeed, every working farm the urbanite passes by on their interstate fly-bys commenced as a dream, an inkling of the possible amid the improbable. Every farm was conceived as a twinkling in the eye, a burning of the ear, a flight of fancy that began, "Hmm, let me see here…"

Open spaces nourish artistry. Give a thoughtful character time and space to think, mix with a country view outside his or her window, add a fertile landscape amenable to cultivation and, voila, you've grown yourself a visionary soul as ripe as an Iowa Brandywine tomato. Recall that Ray Kinsella himself was an ex-Berkeley idealist drifting into an uninspired middle age before destiny quite literally called to him in a cornfield.

Just because history whispers to us when we're hoeing beans, weeding the garden, or washing the dishes doesn't make us nuts our "touched." Indeed, where else in the United States can you find such a sizable a population still living in the same house, working the same acres, or making the same rounds as their parents or grandparents? Anyone who has lived on a Century or Heritage Farm or in an old family house will tell you they sense their forebears around every corner, their voices forever in their ear, and on the wind.

Middle Americans are born makers. Give a rural denizen some time and a little seed money or modest credit line, and they'll come out of the garage, basement, or machine shed six months later, eyes wilding, with something saleable to show for it. It's all the rage to praise the dot.com wonderkids on the coasts as America's ultimate imaginers, but I'll put Middle America's per capita entrepreneurial spirit up against Silicon Valley's any day. Exhibit A: Turning a once nondescript cornfield into a cultural touchstone and cash cow.

Big ideas take large-spirited partners. Those who don't know better like to portray farm men as gruff, tough, go-it-alone, my-way-or-the-highway lone-wolf types. (Think patriarch Larry Cook in *A Thousand Acres*.) But *Field of Dreams* hits nearer to the truth. In the film it's Ray Kinsella who's intuitive, whimsical, impressionable, and creative, while his life partner, Midwest farm girl Annie Kinsella, is unswerving, steady, determined, and fiercely combative when she finds her family's way of life threatened and her husband's dignity taken from him. Take a closer look at rural history and you'll find that the folks in the covered wagons and prairie schooners, those irrepressible sod-busters, life-bringers, seed-sowers and -savers, had pretty much mastered the gender-flip by 1850. For them gender equity was as urgent and practical as putting food on the table.

Granted, *Field of Dreams* isn't perfect movie magic. Despite its genius it indulges too many rural and small-town stereotypes. Witness the deplorable way small-town folks are represented in the PTA, Terence Mann book-banning scene. But its sins are venial, and it comes as near to getting us right, respectfully, as any blockbuster to reach full leaf and tassel in our lifetime.

It's not quite cinematic heaven but it's close, and I for one was honored to be on the Field when the film celebrated its twenty-fifth anniversary on Father's Day weekend, and the generations communed as easily and naturally as ballplayers over a good game of catch. Over the course of that celebratory weekend the press reported the case of a terminally ill father who spent the day playing catch with his adult sons before readying himself to watch the movie on the inflatable screen in centerfield.

Afterward in the guest registry the father wrote, "I can die now," and his son, directly below him: "My father can die now." Their words remind us of how a film experience as special as this one can, with grace and tenderness, reveal life's ultimate plot.

Agrarian Fireworks

Holidays inevitably leave me feeling contemplative, I suppose because the everyone-is-doing-it mentality awakens in me the cultural critic. They cause me to wonder why, exactly, we do what we do when we do it, whether ritual, rite, or well-rationalized obligation. Fourth of July fireworks are like that for me, putting the place-based agrarian in a profoundly confused, even combustible place.

Mine was not a public fireworks display sort of family. In what would no doubt be considered a reversal of the rural gender stereotypes, it was the women in my farm family who seemed most keen on driving the five miles into town to experience the noisy spectacle put on by our local fire department. The men would hem and haw, dragging their feet at the prospect of going to town for the evening. Going to town for anything other than a trip to the local Farm Service Agency, farm co-op, implement dealership, or hardware store meant getting "cleaned up," and getting "cleaned up" was a chore.

If you were a churchgoer, your rural neighbors might have seen you with that slicked-back, just-from-the-shower look on a Sunday morning, but that's about it. Driving in for pyrotechnics meant letting the townies see you squeaky clean—an intimacy typically reserved for one's family. Seeing a farmer freshly showered was a bit like pulling a dripping wet cat from the bathtub; you hardly recognized them.

Neither did the pigs-in-the-chute jockeying for space on the shoulder of the highway appeal to the men in my family. In fact, our entire lifestyle was built around an assiduous avoidance of exactly that kind of cheek-by-jowl craning for a view. Farmers and ranchers are people of unobstructed views, of wide-open vistas, and, as a rule, their vision is downward, groundward.

Much like shell-shocked veterans shy away from big guns and big blasts, farmers spend their lives amid a cacophony of noises intimating danger, and thus develop a sensitive ear, even if, paradoxically, hours on and around machinery have rendered them hard of hearing. As irony would have it the farmer ultimately seeks a condition of silence, in part because theirs is an inherently noisy world. Practically everything they do involves the rumble and whine of an internal combustion engine.

To drive four or five miles into town to see the fireworks, packing yourself in amid the well-lubricated townies shouting for more and bigger, was antithetical to the agrarians of my youth. If they wanted that kind of eardrum-splitting, thrill-seeking mayhem they might just as well have loaded the family up for a heavy metal stadium concert.

The farmer-rancher, of course, bears a complicated relationship to the bombs-bursting-in-air aspect of Independence Day. Historically they have given more of their blood and treasure to war than any other single profession, and this despite a historically isolationist bent. More than likely the farmer knows someone killed or disfigured by a blast, explosion, or fire. On the farm, or at least on our farm, a gun was a thing to be used as a last resort—a specialized tool like any specialized tool to be used rarely and always with particular purpose and precision. Its use entailed no bragging, bombast, or self-congratulation.

The patriot in me loves the Fourth of July, but the agrarian in me, coupled with the fiscal conservative, make me circumspect in that love. When the grand finale is done, and the last of the embers burn themselves out in the twilight sky stretched over the distant fields, I'm glad I went, if only for the shared celebration of our freedoms. Then the post-pyrotechnic silence returns me to that contemplative mood, thinking of the oddities of our rituals—the ways in which we observe them, and expect others to do likewise, without at least wondering why we do them, what (and whose) interests they serve, and what alternatives there may be. The brain that looks for a better way to reach the same desirable end, the problem-solving brain, is, after all, the yeoman's way.

Each year, after the fire department passes the hat for donations to cover the ever-increasing cost of the show they put on, I wonder what else in our collective lives would draw so many of my fellow townsmen and women out in their cars after dark—certainly not community theater, or a tractor pull, or even the bright Friday night lights of high school football. What is it about this midsummer simulation of war that compels us to gather in such large numbers and in such high spirits? In a twenty-first century revision of the iconic line from *Field of Dreams*, you must do more than build it if you want them to come: you must blow it up.

After the night burns down to embers we pull our cars by the hundreds into the narrow two-lane highway in a scene very much like the final shot in the by-now-classic film. We ease forward into the balmy night, our high beams on, searching for the ghosts of gunpowder days and the brave souls who once fought for their freedom.

Part IV:
Politics

Breakaway Agrarian Republics

The farmer-rancher is legendary for his dislike of anarchy. A fox in the proverbial henhouse, disorder is bad for business. Unsurprisingly then, Middle American states with the greatest number of farms—Texas, Iowa, and Missouri lead the pack—rank among those best-known for stable, business-friendly governance. Iowa, in particular, has been a midlands model for middle-of-the-road steady-as-she-goes government, and boasts the longest-serving governor in US history: Terry Branstad. This don't-rock-the-boat maxim explains in large part the enduring agrarian caution against changing horses midstream.

And yet for all the popular notions of farmer domesticity, stability, and predictability the nation's most virulent secessionist movements have lately taken root in the states with the greatest numbers of farms, especially in Texas. A dozen miles down the road from my own farmstead a neighbor of mine recently made TV news for declaring his own secessionist don't-tread-on-me republic in the small town of Wheatland, Iowa.

Following Britain's vote to exit the European Union in June 2016, Branstad was asked to comment on the reinvigorated Texas secession movement, "Texit." The governor was expected to throw water on the secessionist fires burning in the Lone Star State, which several years earlier had garnered enough petition signatures (in excess of 125,000) to merit a stern, paternalistic reminder from the Obama White House that the Founding Fathers who created the nation "did not provide a right to walk away from it."

"No, we are not the European Union. We are the United States of America and this is a unified country," Branstad told reporters at his weekly news briefing, sticking close to the patriotic party line until he surprised the journalists with a caveat: "But we are also a federalist system, and one of the concerns that a lot of people in Texas have, and a lot of people in Iowa have, is that the direction that this country has been going is that we are seeing the states' rights being whittled away by the federal government, by actions of the administration and by the courts. And there is great concern among many states, including people throughout the United States, on that issue."

It was one thing for then-governor of Texas Rick Perry to contemplate secession—Texas had seceded from Mexico in 1836 and from America itself when it joined the Confederacy in 1861—but many observers registered shock when a petition for Iowa secession earned several thousand signatures, though Hawkeyes who knew their history shouldn't have been at all surprised. In the Great Depression the state had played host to what historian Dale Kramer called the first widespread farmer revolt since Shay's Rebellion in the Revolutionary War: the Iowa Cow Wars. There, in my own home county, a militia of five hundred plowmen clashed with sixty-five sheriffs' deputies in violence that eventually resulted in the calling in of more than eighteen hundred Iowa National Guard troops wielding machine guns and bayonets.

In fact, the otherwise stable Midwestern states have a history not only of armed agrarian rebellion but also of would-be secession. In the Civil War agitators in the North and South drew up a so-called Northwest Confederacy to consist of Ohio, Indiana, Michigan, Wisconsin, Minnesota, Illinois and Iowa. Sounding a lot like Iowa's Terry Branstad, Indiana governor Thomas Hendicks remarked in 1862, "The first and highest interest of the Northwest is in the restoration and preservation of the Union, but if the failure and folly and wickedness of the party in power render a Union impossible then the mighty Northwest must take care of herself and her own interests." The idea of a Northwestern Confederacy had the support of many yeoman—and not just because the South and the Midwest—the latter then called the Northwest—shared a core agricultural identity, but also because they shared lucrative trade relationships formed around the metric tons of grain floated down the Mississippi River to southern markets.

Online the question of an Iowa secession, in particular, has occupied internet wonks and futurists for nearly a decade, beginning in 2008 when the website Debate.org hosted an online debate on the topic. There pro-secessionists began with the premise that the federal government was hurting the state; proponents of leaving logged in to offer a litany of supposed advantages awaiting the Hawkeye State should it elect to exit. Fully one third of the state's federal tax revenue, they claimed, was then going toward paying interest on the national debt. Health care for the many senior citizens in the state would improve dramatically with Iowa's departure, one native secessionist argued, pointing out that in the 1960s Iowa had the most efficient health care in the country. "When Medicare was conceived, they applied statewide spending to a specific formula which would regulate the amount of funding increases received each year in each state," he explained. "This formula has punished us for being efficient, in that now Iowa receives the lowest Medicare funds per capita in the country. Our nurses and medical professionals are unable to make as much as they could in bordering states that are benefiting today from being wasteful in the 1960s."

Nearly ten years later in 2017 the question of Iowa's (and Missouri's) secession was raised on the website Quora, the leave-the-union scenario apparently hinging on the state's 2.5 billion bushels of corn (nearly 20 percent of the national corn production) and 12.5 billion pounds of hogs (approximately 35 percent of the national production.) The viability of a breakaway agrarian republic taking root in the land between the Mississippi and Missouri Rivers, contributors pointed out, likely depended on whether or not the secessionist state would be permitted to trade peaceably with its neighbors. "There are two major scenarios that I can think of," secession-minded Nate Wegner wrote. "The first is that Iowa secedes peacefully and relations with the U.S. are friendly. The second is that Iowa secedes violently, although this would most definitely end badly."

The idea that self-employed farmers and ranchers wield disproportionate economic clout, and that they might one day lead a rebellion similar to the Cow Wars in defense of their interests is something more than internet conspiracy theory, as the forty-one-day occupation of Oregon's Malheur National Wildlife Refuge by rural militias loyal to ranchers Ammon and Cliven Bundy attests, or January 2018's reading from a "Declaration of Independence" for the proposed state of New California. In declaring their independence the ruralists behind the creation of an autonomous New California quoted a clause from the US Declaration of Independence: "That, whenever any Form of Government becomes destructive of these ends, it is the Right of the People to alter or to abolish it, and to institute new Government, laying its foundation on such Principles and organizing its Powers in such form, as to them shall seem most likely to affect their Safety and Happiness." Residents of California's most rural counties, the Declaration maintained, had suffered "the long train of abuses and usurpations at the hands of a tyrannical government." As historical precedent and inspiration they cited West Virginia's ideological breakaway from Virginia during the Civil War in 1861 and subsequent admittance into the union as an independent entity in 1863.

Nationwide interest in secession grows apace. An online survey by Reuters in 2014 found that nearly one in four Americans want their state to secede. The percentage desiring to leave was highest—34 percent—in the Southwest, a region that encompassed Texas. Indeed, the idea that a farm or ranching republic could attempt to secede, or, more likely, that a breakaway agrarian region might leave its own state and seek separate admittance into the United States, appears more likely going forward than equitable reconciliation between agrarian and metropolitan regions. Whether it's farm- and ranch-endowed Texas, or California, or even domesticated Iowa, rural revolt may be just around the bend.

The Red Glow of Pyrotechnic Shifts

When the Governor of New Jersey quietly signed a bill to allow the sale and use of some types of consumer fireworks in 2017, it marked a significant rightward shift in the American body politic, though few if any pundits paused to take notice. According to the American Pyrotechnics Association (APA) New Jersey joined eight other states (Kentucky, Utah, New Hampshire, Michigan, New York, Georgia, West Virginia, and Iowa) in lifting restrictions on the sale and use of some types of consumer fireworks since 2011.

That same summer the state of Iowa fell to the legal fireworks juggernaut. The agrarian commonwealth still remembered a windy day in 1931 in the small town of Spencer, where a fire ignited by a sparkler at a local drug store engulfed nearly one hundred buildings and led to an eighty-year statewide ban on aerial fireworks. And yet with little contentious debate legislators approved a bill legalizing the sale and use of commercial grade fireworks in the state in 2017, including bottle rockets and Roman candles. Iowans overwhelmingly agreed with the new law, with nearly two-thirds of the adults surveyed by a Des Moines Register/Mediacom poll in support of legal fireworks. What's fascinating is not that the state finally approved fireworks (polls leading up to the 2017 legalization consistently found a majority of residents in support) but the ways in which the legalization of consumer fireworks may serve as a litmus for more explosive political changes nationally.

The restriction or outright banning of consumer fireworks has long been a fixture in nearly all of the states author Colin Woodard identifies as belonging to "Yankeedom" in his influential book *American Nations*. Indeed, a 2014 *Washington Post* map of the states that heavily restrict or totally ban consumer fireworks looks very much like a map of reliably Blue Yankee states, including at least three located in the Midwest. Five states circa 2014—Illinois, Iowa, Maine, Ohio, and Vermont—allowed only sparklers and/or novelty fireworks, while four (Delaware, Massachusetts, New Jersey, and New York), together accounting for 11.4 percent of the U.S. population, insisted on blanket bans.

Since 2014 New York and New Jersey have both dropped their blanket bans, Iowa has legalized commercial fireworks, and Illinois may soon follow suit. Of the ten reliably Blue states that the *Post* identified in 2014 as banning fireworks altogether or otherwise restricting their citizens to sparklers/novelties, nearly a third (including political battleground states like Iowa, Ohio, and Arizona) turned Red for Donald Trump in the 2016 general election, defying pollsters expectations.

Woodard characterizes the states of Yankeedom as those largely founded by Puritans, and his map of Yankeedom consists in large part of the Northeastern states and the industrial Midwest—areas, he says, that tend to be more comfortable with government regulation and that prize communality and the common good. These are the states most likely in theory to enact laws to protect children and adults from the threat of fire and injury posed by pyrotechnics. Interestingly, Woodard's map of Yankeedom either partly or completely encompasses (in the case of Iowa and New York), or borders on (in the case of New Jersey) states that have recently approved the use of all or some consumer fireworks.

As far back as 2015 political pundits and pulse-takers might have predicted Iowa's surprising vote for Trump in 2016 if only they had looked at the state's move away from its communal Yankee roots to a more Deep South and Wild West embrace of don't-tread-on-me personal liberties, even if, and when, those liberties conflict with perceptions of the common good. When polled in February 2015 more than 54 percent of Iowans favored legalizing fireworks, with 42 percent opposed. More than 60 percent of the men surveyed registered a favorable response to the question of legalization. The poll numbers evidenced a tell-tale Trump-like gender gap, too, with 62 percent of men saying they supported legalizing fireworks compared with only 46 percent of women.

Curiously, while a majority of Iowans were busy telling pollsters they were in favor of a Red-state fixture—the right to buy and explode aerial fireworks—they were simultaneously telling presidential pollsters they favored Clinton over Trump. As of July 12, 2016, the RealClear Politics (RCP) Poll Average in the state found Clinton with a +5.5 percent margin. By the Fall of 2016 the race had tightened to a virtual dead heat, with most forecasts giving Trump a slight edge at best. Few predicted that Trump would ultimately beat Clinton in the Hawkeye State by nearly double digits.

Had Team Clinton followed the fireworks polling they might have predicted the ideological drift rightward well in advance—perhaps even in time to adjust their ground strategy if not set their sails to the new political winds. While feelings about the legalization of fireworks in historically Yankee states are far from a perfect forecaster of political realignments on the ground, they turn out to offer a far more accurate litmus than polls of likely voters.

A map of the United States of Fireworks looks jarringly different now than it did in 2011. And in agrarian states like Iowa that shift may serve as a harbinger of still more explosive political changes to come, and a Red glow likely to linger longer than political forecasters predicted.

When the Government Says Go

Silly. Stubborn. Stupid. Selfish. When I made the decision to defy state and county officials and remain behind fire lines that summer of the Soberanes Fire I heard all those epithets and more. Granted, a 130,000 plus-acre California wildfire is a slower-moving threat than the winds wrapped around a major hurricane, but having personally experienced the should-I-stay-or-should-I-go decision in both, I know all too well the difficult and intensely personal calculus victims face.

As a second round of record-setting wildfires and landslides struck California a year later, armchair observers overlooked what for many victims is an obvious fact: that natural disasters feel like war to those who go through them. And much like war it's not always possible to know how we will react until the fight-or-flight moment brings the battle to our door.

On paper I am a professor who knows well the scholarship of flawed decision-making—the countless studies documenting our inclination to hang on too long to a lost cause or sinking ship; our too-human tendency to lose the forest for the trees when life-altering choice is urgently required of us.

And yet when the moment for evacuation arrived for me during the summer of 2016 I found, to my alarm, that my scholar's knowledge of sound decision-making flew from me in a heartbeat—and that I was no more willing to abandon ship than

I would willingly abandon a family member or a long-time friend in need. The commonsensical advice given otherwise dutiful caretakers of all kinds—save yourself first—is especially hard to follow when the pressure is on and the full fiduciary weight of a caretaker's obligation presses in, conflating emotion with reason and clouding one's judgment. Sometimes warnings from local officials arrive too late; sometimes text alerts are missed by rural residents living off-grid or purposefully unplugged; sometimes palpable fear tricks the uninsured into believing that death is a risk worth taking in order to defend a home that's all they have; that makes life worth living for them. Sometimes conditions on the ground deteriorate swiftly and without warning.

Otherwise rational observers watching coverage of natural disasters on television tell themselves they would surely have heeded official warnings, gotten the hell out and played it safe. And yet whether a would-be victim of a natural disaster stays or goes, experience has taught me, is as individual and idiosyncratic as end-of-life health care decisions, and far from one size fits all. The poor, the uninsured, the immigrant, the aged and elderly, the sick, the solitary, the deeply spiritual and rural rooted—all face a uniquely different set of variables as they weigh the ultimate decision. Those who have never faced an order to leave a home cannot fully comprehend with what terrifying speed the dominos fall.

That summer I told worried friends and family members that I was ready to die in order to defend the uninsured remote cabin where I was staying. I felt big and bold when making these declarations, and strangely final, though the true finality of death would surely have left me begging for my life.

I confess that the ideologue in me stopped more than once to admire the certainty in these live-free-or-die sentiments, foolish and dangerous as they were. While I was fairly sure that the cabin, tucked away beneath a canopy of trees, could not be seen by the helicopters dropping fire retardant, and wholly certain that it could not be reached by fire tanker up the steep mountain road, it should have been readily apparent that the cabin was not worth my life; my plan, I said, was to keep the roof and wood siding wet when the fire drew near with a combination of the garden hoses used on the property for irrigation and a single fire hose that lay curled up out back like the shed skin of a very large snake. At the time this seemed like a plan that could reasonably be executed; a creeping fire ignited by a random ember could sometimes be put out before igniting the rest of the structure. But the Soberanes was not a spot fire; I could see its forty-foot-plus eruptions of flame marching inexorably toward me from miles away.

Only after the danger of fire had passed—coming within a mile of where I kept my stubborn and stupid vigil—did I stop to consider how deeply rooted in agrarian values my decision to stay behind had been. Ignoring evacuation orders reflected my deep-seated distrust of government mandates and dictates. I had not trusted the county sufficiently to sign up for the emergency text system made available to residents and seasonal visitors like me. I had not filled out the paperwork left behind by the local fire departments asking for information about the location of propane tanks and persons on the property; presumably to pre-identify risk and, posthumously, bodies. In truth I had not completed the paperwork because, tucked behind several cattle gates in the mountains and largely inaccessible, the cabin had been missed by the leafletting.

Still, as the fire drew near the daytime skies darkened and ash floated down from the heavens in a firescape that can only be described as apocalyptic, I grew anxious enough to hand-paint my own sign and lay it down in the front pasture, print-side up, so that the tankers and helicopters carrying water and retardant to the fire might know I was there. The purity of my principled idiocy had been reduced to something shy of 100 percent as the possibility of my own demise became more imminent.

My decision to value the welfare of the land over my own safety reached back to my agricultural roots, to the men and women I grew up with who would do anything to maintain their property rights, keep their land from bankers and government officials, or otherwise preserve their autonomy as lords of their particular barnyards. As a boy such love sometimes seemed obsessive to me; a mad lust or land-love driven beyond reason by a passion that would throw even immediate family members under the bus if the sanctity of the home acres was threatened. A disregard for one's own health and well-being, a fatalistic interest in the very Acts of God—fire, tornado, flood—that had the power to humble man or woman; these too were part of my agrarian inheritance.

During the nights when I would sit in the cabin's loft to watch the five-story-tall flames approach, my anxious thoughts returned to childhood images of my father and grandfather leaving the safety of the basement on our Midwestern farm to watch as a funnel clouds or tornadoes neared, while the women in the family called loudly for them to stop being fools, to come back inside where it was safe. Though frightening, their willingness to stay behind in the path of what seemed certain destruction seemed heroic to me, though later I would come to see the selfishness in it, too. While the women and children in our family were directed to safety the men granted themselves agency and choice in the face of disaster. If they wanted to die they would die; the rest of us would survive whether we liked it or not.

It was a poor message to send to children, but in the intervening years I have grown to see it more ambivalently, too, for in bucking conventional wisdom they were also teaching valuable lessons about courage, about self-reliance, about insisting on seeing Death yourself, and about living and dying by the same sword if necessary. The calculus of their moral equations was and is difficult to simply or unequivocally comprehend.

Experiencing a 130,000-acre wildfire taught me that when it comes to natural disasters otherwise good and rational people make impossibly difficult decisions given unique circumstances whose philosophical, practical, ideological and spiritual complexities cannot be fully understood by those watching on television. Those of us lucky enough to survive nature's calamities know better than to make heroes of those who stay behind. But we know too that often the last-ditch, lost-cause decision to defend an endangered home is in many ways a noble impulse.

Granted, ignoring or being ignorant of emergency orders is foolish. But before we yield to our too-human tendency to blame the stubbornness of the stayers-behind or those who left too late, we should remember the empathetic principle—that faced with the exigencies of emergency and the fight-or-flight of a war come unbidden to our door, "they" might well have been us.

New Crops and Old Worries

Not so long ago I found myself spending the summer living adjacent to two nascent California mid-coast marijuana farms. As irony would have it I had landed in the Golden State at a time when recreational and medicinal weed were on the ballot in states across the nation. As California and eight other states readied themselves to vote on loosening their marijuana laws, my neighbor thrilled at the prospect of legalized weed, a crop he called "the next wine grape."

I met him in the way most rural folks do: over the fence. He's a husband, father, and landowner. He seemed understandably sensitive about his property being used to grow medical marijuana, though perhaps not as sensitive as the family that had, up until recently, been renting the house on his property. The renters had overreacted, he explained, to the unannounced late-night visits of the licensed marijuana grower who was using the far reaches of the land unbeknownst to the renters. Apparently the tenants had reported the operation to the county sheriff. A stink had ensued but no consequences had come of it, the sheriff being too busy, the neighbor said, to enforce the law. The only real result of the reported violation had been that the tenant, a concerned parent of three small children and a recent out-migrator from Los Angeles, had immediately moved back to the coast, threatening a lawsuit over the remaining lease, not wanting to subject her kids to the culture of the crop that was growing in the field below her rural rental, right under her nose.

Concerned, I suppose, that I would be the prototypical stick-in-the-mud who might throw a wrench in his plans, the neighbor kindly offered to show me the grower's license to cultivate medical marijuana, though the volume of cannabis being grown, so far as I could tell, was far in excess of what could reasonably be used medically by a single individual or family. I kept whatever objections I may have had mostly to myself, trying to buy his "new wine grape" rationale, though inside I found myself wondering. And having myself spent a fair amount of time in some of the California's best-known wine grape regions—Napa and Sonoma, Paso Robles, Carmel Valley—I wasn't entirely sure I bought his premise. Wine grapes have been a boon not just to rural economies but to arts, culture, and community in the countryside. Despite their perceived elitism, tasting rooms, cafes, gifts shops, and free or low-cost events put on by vineyard and winery owners often bring stakeholders together to find common cause, while simultaneously attracting visitors and new residents. Perhaps the same will be true of legalized pot, though the verdict is still out.

I had happily rented in the area once before, though that summer, marred by raging wildfires and evacuations, turned out to be a far cry from a vacation. Many illegal growers in the rugged mid-coast mountains lost their crops in the conflagrations—some, as reported by major media, actually fired their guns at the fire personnel trying to save them—but so far as I know my neighbor's crop thrived in the unusually warm, smoky conditions. His grower made it behind fire lines to nurse the precious buds through the period of greatest danger, and by the end of my summer in the cabin the smell of weed in bloom infused the air for miles, penetrating upholstery and clothes indoors and out with its uniquely pungent odor. Its stench infiltrated everything, so much so that when I offered acquaintances a lift into town, I was certain they would, taking a whiff of the car seats, confuse me for yet another Gen X pothead. Something of a goody two-shoes by comparison with my peers elsewhere in Legalization Nation, I was powerfully and probably needlessly self-conscious about this.

I thought about the neighbor's erstwhile renter—the mom who moved her family far away rather than expose her children to the marijuana culture. Had she been a stick-in-the-mud, or had she merely known that living next to cash-crop agriculture on even a small scale is enough to cause many urbanites and suburbanites to reconsider rural living. We know this phenomenon all too well back home in the rural Heartland—metropolitan drop-outs coming to live, cheek by jowl, across from multi-generational farms like the one owned by my family—and inevitably objecting to the sounds and the smells of our culture: agriculture.

Not being a smoker myself, I can't claim to understand marijuana culture intuitively, nor can I claim to know how rural life in states like California will change once and if marijuana becomes the next wine grape. But I do know it will change, and change significantly. I understand from experience that commodity-crop agriculture alters a community and a region in ways those voting on legalization ought to consider. Unlike in the Midwest and Mid-South, where we mostly harvest our cash crops ourselves, the cannabis crop in California seems likely to be harvested and grown, plantation-style, by someone other than the well-to-do property owner, as is often the case with the wine grape. The marijuana property owner, in effect, acts as patron of the hacienda, hiring workers to do their bidding. This means paid growers, paid harvesters, and the steady stream of visitors—mostly from city to country—wanting to enjoy some homegrown on-site. It also often means exponentially larger water usage and sometimes strained relations in communities where growers and non-growers share fence-lines, roads, and wells.

Whatever the decision on legalization in their home states, folks living in cities, suburbs, and exurbs should consider the Not-in-my-back-yard (NIMBY) phenomenon as it relates to marijuana growing. And if they would object to the smells, the suspicions, the increased water usage, the late-night visits, the hacienda and patron system cropping up in their own quiet cul-de-sacs and gated communities, they might more carefully consider their ballot. To vote Yes with integrity, America's metropolitan voters would want to walk a mile in their country cousins' shoes, imagining whether, if, and to what extent, they would be comfortable living across the fence from this potent "new" agriculture.

Savoring Straw Polls

Critics argue that presidential straw polls of the kind recently held in Iowa, Illinois, and New Hampshire are expensive and a poor predictor of candidate viability. I, however, find the straw poll's charms many and alluring, so long as one appreciates them for what they are: political pomp and spectacle mixed with old-fashioned picnic populism.

I attended my first presidential straw poll in Ames, Iowa, in 2011 and came away convinced of its ultimate utility. What was then the nation's most famous political scrimmage easily represented the best chance citizens had to meet the entire slate of GOP presidential candidates. And isn't that the point? To let folks size up the job applicants in the flesh and on the hoof, serving as a sort of well-fed focus group?

And yet to hear the national media tell it the straw poll is an exercise in shameless pandering. Democratic strategist Edward Kilgore claimed in the pages of *Salon* that it had needlessly lengthened the campaign season and "complicated the lives of candidates and their strategists, who are forced either to propitiate or defy the Corn Idol months before the first real votes are cast." Brian Montopoli of CBS News one-upped Kilgore's rant in an article uncharitably entitled "An absurd, candidate-killing spectacle returns," wherein he floated his own diatribe: "The Iowa Straw Poll is something of a fraudulent affair, an alleged test of candidate support in which votes are bought and Iowans are bribed to attend with free barbecue and entertainment."

Critics inevitably pile on, but even as they rail, chances for the kind of face-to-face flesh-pressing and feet-to-the-flame-questioning offered by straw polls grow rarer with each election cycle. What makes straw polls so unique is that they happen in real-time, staged in an outdoor mall of sorts where the candidates bid on space in what amounts to a lucrative political fundraiser for the state party rather than for individual candidates. Staffers spend days customizing and planning the retail-political space on which they have successfully bid, turning each into a kind of boutique shop where their candidate is the exclusive product on offer.

Voters are the beneficiary of this mad scramble for walk-in-traffic, wending their way through the various candidate tents as they might amble down a state fair midway, or, more accurately, stroll from house to house at a progressive party. Would-be electors can sample what Candidate A offers before moseying a few doors down to sample the goodies proffered by Candidate B, and so on. The straw poll makes voters feel as if the candidates for president are more like new neighbors on the block than professional politicians—neighbors who've invited them over for heavy hors d'oeuvres and light political conversation. Now, with the demise of state party-sanctioned straw polls, presidential candidates can, with a combination of strategic ad buys, well-placed surrogates, and savvy use of social media, make it seem as if they're in-house when they're actually halfway across the country. Not so at the straw poll, where a missing candidate is as gauche as a host who invites you to dinner only to turn up AWOL when it's time to sling the hash.

National political bosses condescend to the homely straw poll and the contrarian or unconventional candidates it sometimes elevates primarily because they can't control how voters will act on that single fateful day when the non-binding votes are cast and the tallies are broadcast by a headline-hungry national news media. Will voters be more impressed with Candidate A's political chops and gratis pulled pork sandwich, or Candidate B's cool hard logic and complimentary soft ice cream? In a straw poll members of the electorate might be swayed by ethos, pathos, logos, or Cheetos.

On television party bosses and TV pundits laugh at the barbecue stains on voter bibs and sneer at just how easily and cheaply the *demos* is plied for their votes with cheap plastic giveaways and greasy food. And yet the party bosses' inability to predict the results of the day's vote is precisely why reinstituting straw polls would be a boon to old-fashioned agrarian populism. We the People use straw polls to our advantage in an era when candidates otherwise prefer to meet on *their* terms—carefully scripted in cyberspace, on television, or in social media—rather than on our turf. And if candidates for president want to treat us to beef brisket or barbecue ribs, we shouldn't be portrayed as dupable simpletons if we accept. At the straw poll the tables are turned, and it's the candidate's job to play gracious host rather than fly-by-night exploitative guest. We the People do the interviewing, not some talking head on television.

So if you're on the fence about whether America's grassroots states should revive the straw poll in the next presidential election, I say give it a chance. Love it or hate it, at least it's homegrown.

The Plot of Grassroots Politics

Each and every Caucus season I am fortunate to attend an endless panoply of campaign events. This is the lucky lot of an Iowan—citizenship's Golden Ticket.

Imagine the boon—an underpopulated agrarian state of approximately three million people has since 1972 selected the presumptive frontrunner in the contest to be the next leader of the Free World. What novelist could dream up such a plot? It's a premise sufficiently whimsical that not even the most daring filmmaker could storyboard it—something akin to cooking up a plot whereby Lithuania or Latvia is granted the privilege of selecting the next leader of the United Nations. And of course the Hawkeye State's political pole position is rife with irony, as Iowa long ago ceased to be representative of an increasingly diverse, non-white, urban nation.

No wonder, then, that the Caucuses threaten to explode, literally and figuratively, each and every four years, as competing states threaten to leapfrog the first-in-the-nation status and protest groups plan to disrupt the vote. In many ways Caucus night has taken on the drama and suspense inherent in Carnival, with Mardi Gras-like potential for mishap and misadventure. It's a drama the Republication National Committee learned to fear in 2012, when election officials wrongly declared Mitt Romney the winner, then months later certified Rick Santorum the victor in the ultimate plot twist.

Or consider 2016, when Senator Ted Cruz's campaign left recorded messages with Iowans promulgating the "breaking news" that Ben Carson would drop out of the race, urging them to "inform any Carson caucus-goers of this news and urge them to caucus for Ted instead." The *New York Times* outed not only the eleventh-hour effort made by the Cruz campaign to delude the populous but also the text of the fraudulent call, which read: "Hello, this is the Cruz campaign with breaking news: Dr. Ben Carson will be suspending campaigning following tonight's caucuses." Cruz ultimately carried the Caucuses in what amounted to a denouement, but earned the nickname "Lyin' Ted" for his campaign's alleged dirty tricks.

While politically damning for the GOP such skullduggery is ripe for the political novelist. Dramatic reversals and plot twists enhance the built-in irony of the campaign narrative. And perhaps the biggest irony of all is this: Presidential candidates that increasingly do not hail from small Middle American hamlets and villages arrive from the monied coasts feeling the pressing need to present themselves as experts in agricultural policy. The rhetorical exigency lends grotesquerie and buffoonery to the process, as men and women who have neither reaped nor sown attempt to impress the salt-of-the-earth yeomen and yeowomen they presume make up the majority of their audience. Instead, statistics say that would-be voters at any campaign stop in the Hawkeye State are more likely to work in finance, real estate, or insurance than on the farm. According to the raw employment data they are seven or eight times more likely to be working in government or manufacturing than they are plowing a furrow.

In a state that's flipped from rural to urban in the last half century (Iowa is now nearly 65 percent urban), many once agrarian small towns have turned into de facto bedroom communities where America's iconic small-town residents no longer know their neighbors. Most do their shopping in the nearest university town rather than at home on Main. As a result the surprising assemblage of Caucus-goers who gather on election night remains a mystery until the very last minute, like an Agatha Christie novel wherein the suspects arrive one by one to reveal their identities. Every four years small-town denizens who once routinely encountered one another at the local grocery store, bank, or city hall, now caucus with neighbors they've never even seen before. Like a Western (or a Middle Western) no one knows who's going to walk through the doors of the local community center or fire hall to cast their lot. Whoever they are, though, it's a good bet they'll be welcomed at the ballot box. In some of the state's smallest precincts election officials still make popcorn on an old stove while voters debate their votes out in the hall.

The Caucus season is sufficiently long, at six or seven months from the state fair in August to Groundhog Day in early February, as to lend itself to the rising action the novelist seeks, replete with plot twists as the allegiances (and suspicions) of a fickle electorate flow from this candidate to that and back again in the suspenseful advent to election eve. As a consequence the Hawkeye State's role in the presidential nomination process has gone from salt-of-the-earth presidential predictor to apple-cart-upsetter and advancer of underdog or insurgent candidates—from Rick Santorum's after-the-fact win in 2012 to Barack Obama's surprising drubbing of Hillary Clinton in 2008 to Donald Trump's unexpectedly strong polling in 2016.

In the end the imaginative writer recognizes in Iowa's peculiar corn poll not only an enduring American folkway but also a fragile and vulnerable political tradition needing saving. And because national party bosses decide who stands at the front of the line each election season, Iowa's status as first-in the-nation is very much in jeopardy, especially after the embarrassing vote-counting gaffs of 2012. In a world where digitally-powered populism increasingly stands at odds with political party king-makers manipulating public perception, the state's days as presidential bellwether and harbinger must surely be numbered.

For, bye and bye, we have begun to think independently, meaning that we have become what many power-hungry party elites have good reason to fear: a highly literate, well-educated, semi-rural *demos* with few external barriers to participation—a citizenry with the time, inclination, ability, and mobility to hear the candidates in person and to decide for ourselves.

When—not if—the primacy of the state's stand-alone first-in-the-nation vote is threatened, redemptive acts of voter-centered imagining and re-imagining, coupled with well-reasoned arguments for why such a cultural folkway should matter to the rest of the nation, stand the best chance of keeping the long-running political drama going strong.

Family Business Is Not Necessarily Nepotism

Ever since the uproar over Ivanka Trump's sitting in for her father at the "adult's table" at the G20 summit in Hamburg, Germany, I've been thinking about why it is that we seem so eager to cry nepotism where family enterprises are concerned. The pundits positively erupted at the sight of Ivanka seated between the British prime minister and the Chinese president. Foreign policy wonk Brian Klass denounced the image of the "unelected, unqualified, daughter-in-chief" while others sneered at Trump's self-styled "take-your-daughter-to-work day."

I don't share the sense of righteous indignation at one trusted family member ceremonially standing in for another for an afternoon. Maybe it's because I grew up in the small-town Midwest, a place where parent-child businesses have been the norm for generations. At home on the farm, on a shelf handmade by my grandfather, sits my great-grandfather's *Account Book and Farm Record*. On the inside cover great-grandpa has written "Business Record of W.T. Jack & Son, Breeders of Hampshire Hogs, Record starting Jan 1. 1922." I do the math and realize my great-grandfather declared his son a business partner two weeks after his son's 5th birthday. Their business motto: "We eat what we can't sell."

The fevered pitch of the attacks against The Donald and The Daughter give the cultural critic in me pause: What is it, exactly, that certain segments of America find so frightening about such close parent-child bonds, be they in business or politics (and isn't politics a business?) Do they feel threatened by family business because urban America has so completely promulgated the myth of meritocracy—that the person best able to do the job gets the job? Or is it the mere existence of qualities such as trust and loyalty that are *not* ascertainable via academic credentials that irk urban professionals and policy wonks, especially in a world where professionals rack up tens of thousands of dollars of debt to buy degrees they believe will increase their chances of getting hired instead of the "inside," "in-house," or "family" candidate?

Granted, the world leaders who attended the G20 summit have the right to be disappointed at the elevation of the First Daughter to the high-level table, in much the same way that, in hiring father/son plumbers, one naturally hopes to have the more experienced father on the wrench, though let's be honest: the seasoned hand is not always the most expert or up-to-date. But do Chicago and the rest of the metro Midwest, places built on tightly knit and often reputable family businesses, have the right to such righteous indignation? At root I suspect the vilification of so-called nepotism is, like so much in our culture, a geopolitical phenomenon.

In the agrarian Midwest, Ivanka's stint in her father's stead is widely regarded as a testament of her father's faith in his daughter-adviser as understudy, and as an affirmation of her father's family-first loyalties put into practice. In other more technocratic metropolitan ZIP codes where the bias against family enterprise is deeply lodged, the veneration of the impartial expert over trusted kin or close associate may explain the outrage with which President Trump's move was received. In either case the strength of feeling on both sides of the "Ivankagate" debate makes sense. It's yet another example of two Americas: one comforted by tradition, the other alarmed and offended by tradition's reliance on inner circles.

In a highly mobile business world where education and paper credentials are expected to trump homegrown knowledge, on-the-ground connections, and familial ties, the cultural tensions at the heart of the First Daughter's priority seating will linger on long after she has left the table.

Political Epistles

In 1924 my great-aunt Mary Puffer, later to become Mary Brown, won the handsome sum of fifteen dollars put up by a Mechanicsville, Iowa, consortium of businesspeople and local politicians for the best open letter about the town submitted to the local newspaper, the *Pioneer Press*. In declaring Mary the prizewinner for her letter entitled "A Perfect Community," the Contest Committee wrote that they had a "bunch of good letters" but that one stood out. "The following letter," the Committee noted, "indicates a keen mind, close observation, and a fine mental attitude toward the home community." And either to register disbelief, to drive home a point, or both, the Committee added, "And it was written by a young person."

Mary passed away before I had a chance to ask her about her intentions for her award-winning missive of long-ago, but I believe she wrote in earnest. Her hometown was indeed a bustling place back in those days, fortuitously located on the coast-to-coast Lincoln Highway and the Chicago Northwestern rail line. Surely she intended no exaggeration when she wrote, "I think it is possible to have a perfect community—at least a community as nearly perfect as anything has ever been." Back then Mechanicsville boasted its own opera house and the famed Page Motel, where Bob Hope and other Golden Age stars overnighted as they sojourned across the country. And yet a mere sixty-five years after Mary caught the ears of our city fathers with her lyrical lines, journalist Osha Gray Davidson published *Broken Heartland: The Rise of America's Rural Ghetto*, a book that opened with a chapter-length case study on Mary's hometown and mine. According to Davidson the place had gone from riches to rags in the intervening six decades.

Or had we, its citizens?

Grant me this chicken-and-egg argument: Is it the laudatory letter—the poetry of a place written in prose—that in the minds of reader-citizens reinforces the idea of a perfect community, or the perfect community that inspires and elicits such a laudatory letter? Do towns like mine and Mary's devolve into so-called rural ghettos because they are no longer capable of inspiring lofty and laudatory language, or because the town's boosters and defenders have yielded to complacency and surrendered the ability to be inspired—to be so moved? What happens when a town loses its homegrown poets, those most able to see and express the overlooked potential of the homey and homely? In a nutshell the question is this: who's to blame when love ends, the one who stops writing love letters or the one who is no longer sufficiently lovable to merit gushing recitations? It's my belief that letters have the power to transform our relationships with one another and with the place we live, inasmuch as a letter alone can begin a courtship, sustain it, and end it.

Iowa, in particular, has produced more than its fair share of well-known letter-writers and advice-givers, including two of the most famous American advice columnists, Ann Landers and Abigail Van Buren (of "Dear Abby" fame) from Sioux City. To begin at the beginning of Midwestern letters, however, one must start with the original Henry Wallace, scion of the famous political family that would go on to produce a future Secretary of Agriculture and a Vice-President of the United States. "Uncle Henry," as he came to be known, prided himself on being on a familiar basis with the loyal readers of his *Wallaces' Farmer*, and he made no attempt to disguise the moralizing propaganda he practiced in his letters to region's rural and small-town young people, appending the name "Uncle Henry's Sermons" to the epistles he wrote for *Wallaces' Farmer*. In one such collection, *Letters to the Farm Boy*, Wallace explains to an imagined farmer's son his qualifications for lecturing: "Your Uncle Henry is now over sixty years old, and can, therefore talk to you as he would not have dared to do twenty years ago." In another letter on the subject of a farm boy and his temper, the elder Wallace writes, "My Dear Boy: I have not sized you up as goody-goody.... Such boys are too often like the apples that ripen too early, indicating that the tree is on the decline." Like his fellow agrarian Teddy Roosevelt, who once declared, "I ask nothing of the nation except that it so behave as each farmer here behaves with reference to his own children," Wallace viewed it as a political and cultural necessity for America's farm children to stay put on the farm.

Another well-known agrarian tempted into the politics of epistolary advice-giving was Isaac Phillips Roberts, who moved to Iowa in 1862 with his young bride to take up farming in Mount Pleasant. Roberts proved a quick study as an agrarian, and before the decade was up he had been hired as a superintendent of the farm and secretary of the board of trustees of the newly formed Iowa Agricultural College at Ames, later to become Iowa State University. In his book *The Fertility of the Land* Roberts, like Wallace, invents a composite farm boy to serve as a conversational foil in a chapter titled "A Chat with a Young Farmer":

> I am well-acquainted with you, though you are not acquainted with me, and being acquainted and older than you are, I cannot forbear entering into a little familiar chat. I know your thoughts, your toils and sorrows and discouragements; your aspirations, hopes and joys. I know, too, what fiber, endurance and patience farm work gives to the boys who make the most of what an outdoor life with nature has to offer. I know how hot it is in August under the peak of the flat-roofed barn, how large the forkfuls are that the stalwart pitcher thrusts into the only hole where light and air can enter. I know how high the thistles grow, and how far the rows of corn stretch out. I know, too, the freedom, fun and work of the old farm that make one expand, enjoy and grow, and leave no bitter memories. I know you well…—how green and brown you feel when you come to the noisy city, and how you would like to be free and cool again!

Reading Roberts it's easy to see how quickly the invitation to provide intergenerational advice turns the advice-giver into barnyard philosopher and politician. And yet Roberts surely writes as much for himself as for his youthful readers. To pretend otherwise of an open letter—that is, that its audience is not as much the writer themselves—is to deny its singular rhetorical power. Where else but in such bully pulpit letters do we find ourselves so genuinely warm of heart and pure of intention and at the same time so shamelessly transparent in advancing our political and cultural arguments?

When my Aunt Mary ascended the makeshift stage to receive her fifteen-dollar prize from the Contest Committee, she was, the *Pioneer Press* reported, "profusely applauded" for her pro-hometown propaganda. Aunt Mary had discovered for herself the virtue and the vice of the open letter—its sweet sincerity on one hand, and its cringe-worthy presumptions on the other. It makes an ironic kind of sense that Midwesterners would be both the nation's most prolific writers of advice letters, and its most willing and forthcoming moralizers and propogandists of place. Whether due to our religion-derived talent for judgement and criticism of others, or our defining geo-demographic predicament, which finds older rural Americans circumstantially more apt to write wish-you-were here missives to youthful leave-takers and Brain-Drainers, we have, almost by accident, cultivated extraordinary epistolary gifts. By dint of practice we find ourselves far better at giving advice to the rest of a restless and roving nation than we are at receiving counsel and critique from those who dare to write back.

Years ago I finally succumbed to the regional temptation, agreeing to solicit and edit a collection of advice letters written to the region's young people by its most established luminaries and VIPs. Over the course of twelve months I received, edited, and anthologized hundreds of such missives penned by Governors, Olympians, Poets Laureate, and everything in between—good, caring, civic-minded people who wanted nothing more, in the end, than to see the next generation live well and prosper in the shared place they called home. I confess I finished the project buoyed by the support and nurture I felt bubbling up between the lines like a wellspring.

Still, a cautionary note must be sounded regarding the limitations of even the most well-meaning intergenerational open letters, wherein the old presume to advise the young. And still more needs to be said about the virtues of such an honest and forthright enterprise. Deeply ambivalent at the prospect, I leave the difficult task to another famed Midwestern moralizer and newspaper columnist, the Ohio-born writer Sherwood Anderson and his short story collection *Winesburg, Ohio*:

> The old man had listed hundreds of the truths in his book. I will not try to tell you of all of them. There was the truth of virginity and the truth of passion, the truth of wealth and of poverty, of thrift and of profligacy, of carelessness and abandon. Hundreds and hundreds were the truths and they were all beautiful.... It was the truths that made the people grotesques. The old man had quite an elaborate theory concerning the matter. It was his notion that the moment one of the people took one of the truths to himself, called it his truth, and tried to live his life by it, he became a grotesque and the truth he embraced became a falsehood. You can see for yourself how the old man, who had spent all of his life writing and was filled with words, would write hundreds of pages concerning this matter. The subject would become so big in his mind that he himself would be in danger of becoming a grotesque. He didn't.... It was the young thing inside him that saved the old man.

Too Old to Rock and Roll, but Young Enough to Protest

"Too old to rock and roll, too young to die," went one of my late father's favorite sayings. Dad was paraphrasing that flute-wielding '60s politico Jethro Tull, who had prophesied the great middle-age ennui that would overtake the Boomers when they grew long enough in the tooth to begin collecting social security.

American Boomers are widely considered the wealthiest generation the world has ever known, leaving economists and financial planners wondering what such a cultural force of nature would ultimately spend its collective nest egg on. Would well-off Boomers buy for their fortunate sons the infamous "dude houses" that have recently made headlines in hip Midwestern college towns? Would they pony up their hard-earned dollars for watercolor-worthy coastal or mountain real estate, as they have in recent years when second homes accounted for 40 percent of home sales?

Or would they instead resurrect mothballed traditions for civic engagement in college towns turned retirement meccas such as Madison or Ann Arbor or Iowa City—the latter given laurels as a *Money* magazine best place to retire. And would they return to wearing Birkenstocks, watching indie films, and coming in late reeking of smoky merlot, reliving the cultural experiment that was their college years?

The Occupy Wall Street movement gave America an inkling of what was possible when Boomers left the Pottery Barn and Pier One for the dens of protest. In college towns across the nation gray-hairs donned caps bearing slogans such as "Grannys for a Livable Future" and sweaters that proudly proclaimed "Grandmas for Peace." Regardless of your political bent the potential mobilization of the nation's swell of senior citizens made America stand up and pay attention. Imagine the civic-topia created by a people trading in their AARP cards to renew long-expired political licenses. Fancy a generation dumping its 401-Ks for bully pulpits, taking to council chambers and boards of supervisors for a real-life exam in Politics 101. The Midwest's future would be forever changed, and so would America's.

If the marches of the Occupy movement were indeed a harbinger of political sea-change to come and not just a flash in the generational pan, there might just be some truth in Lewis Mumford's notion that every generation revolts against its fathers and makes friends with its grandfathers. In Occupy protests 20-something-year-old protestors held megaphones for mad-as-hell Boomers old enough to be their grandparents.

My friend Kevin, a grandpa, wrote me a letter recently in which he blew the whistle on his own agemates. "The generation-that-can't-quite-get-over-its-bad-self," he wrote, "has almost put the finishing touches on a culture of total make-believe, where all you have to do is make the minimum payment, where you can indeed get something for nothing. . . ." Initially Kevin's sentiments struck me as so many sour grapes, but now I see in them a reminder that Boomers, the eldest of whom are now well into their seventies, have the collective power to turn a wayward ship of state. It's safe to say grandparents have the potential to do for the rest of the country what they have long done for their families and for rural American communities: remind We the People of the better angels of our natures.

So, if your favorite silver-haired candidate breaks your heart at the voting booth this upcoming election season, take heart. Ask your grandparents to the presidential ball instead. They're likely to surprise you with the moves they know—the pre-Facebook Grapevine, the Electoral Slide, and that timeless and inspiring classic, the Election Year Twist.

Color Me Purple

In an era when America increasingly divides itself into red and blue, I'm privileged to come from a purple state.

Of mostly Welsh and English extraction, my paternal ancestors typify the settlement patterns described in author Colin Woodard's intriguing book *American Nations: A History of the Eleven Rival Regional Cultures of North America*. Woodard maps a wider region he calls "Yankeedom" that stretches from Long Island, New York, all the way to Scott County, Iowa, where my Yankee ancestor Levi Pickert first disembarked in 1854 looking for good land. Yankeedom, Woodard writes, is the product of a Puritan legacy seeking a "perfect earthly society via social engineering," individual mastery of temptation, and a "vigorous government to thwart would-be tyrants."

Pre-Civil War, the regional culture of Yankeedom ended almost exactly at Scott County, Iowa, where another rival regional culture began, ideologically analogous yet distinct. Traveling on foot west to adjacent Cedar County to arrive at what would become our heritage farm, Levi Pickert unwittingly crossed into an entirely new "nation" in Woodard's lexicon: "The Midlands," a long yet narrow swath of counties following good loam from Philadelphia to roughly Lincoln, Nebraska. Woodard defines the Midlands as "culturally pluralistic," a place founded by English Quakers who were less consumed with "ethnic and religious purity" than with affirming their community-minded creed. My Quaker paternal great-great-great grandparents, the Jacks, fit the bill exactly, settling in the one of the largest Quaker communities west of the Mississippi River in West Branch, Iowa, where they happily neighbored with Herbert Hoover's family. To apply Woodard's historical taxonomy to the present day, it's fair to say that when one lives in Cedar County, Iowa, as my family has for seven generations, one lives on the edge of an invisible but all-important geo-cultural fissure, a Middle American ideological equivalent of the Continental Divide.

Woodard bases his map on historical migration patterns dating back to the Colonial period—tracking the routes by which culturally distinct settlers moved West in well-traveled paths—though his historical lens proves uncannily contemporary. If one accepts his premise on faith—that the Midlands region of the Middle West and Great Plains serves as "physical and political buffer between rival regions" such as the far Yankee North and Greater Appalachia Mid-South, it stands to reason that this geographical and cultural middle ground would register the sort of political friction known to produce purple politics. As a result of hosting the very fault line that runs between distinct Yankeedom and Midlands regional cultures, eastern Iowa, in particular, would be colored deep purple in an election as ideologically split as 2016's, as historically disparate cultures ground against one another with near tectonic force.

Until Trump v. Clinton split the popular vote and divided America, I was tempted to dismiss maps like Woodard's as mostly abstract overlays or mere academic takes on political differences underlying Middle America. But the 2016 polling data largely substantiated the geo-demographical fault line Woodard dared to delineate. In 2016 the small town of Wyoming, in Jones County, Iowa, where I drink my coffee at the local café and fill up my tank at the Casey's general store, made headlines as "the most purple of all Iowa cities." In an article titled "The Lone Iowa town in a Political Dead Heat" Mike Kilen of the *Des Moines Register* describes my local whistle stop as "politically purple as they come" with exactly one hundred and fifty-two registered Democrats and one hundred and fifty-two registered Republicans. In fact, three of the state's five "most purple cities" (Wyoming, Wheatland, and Olin) were located in Cedar and Jones County, places whose eastern borders precisely traced Woodard's Yankeedom-Midlands fault line from long ago.

I might have been tempted to dismiss the mantle of "most purple city" as just another election-year novelty story had I not been struck by a similar bolt of statistical lightning in the 2000 general election. At that time I was working as a reporter for a family-run newspaper in the seat of Cedar County, Tipton, Iowa, while covering a Bush-Gore race so close the Supreme Court ultimately decided its outcome. In 2000 Cedar County, where my family had lived since Levi Pickert broke the prairie, was reported to be the only county in the nation to have returned an even draw—4025 for Bush and 4025 for Gore.

In the wake of the tie-vote the national news media descended on our humble offices like a plague of hungry locusts. Now, instead of rubbing shoulders with the alley cats out back, we found ourselves sharing donuts with national correspondents. Cedar County, Iowa, the press declared, was a "national bellwether," a veritable "petri dish of electoral politics." Since

1992, the media discovered, my native agrarian county of just under twenty thousand residents not only backed the winner in each presidential race, but also reflected the statewide general election results. Including its predilection for also backing the winner of the U.S. Senate elections, Cedar County was a perfect 13-and-0 leading up to the election of 2016, when it once again picked the presidential winner, giving the Trump-Pence ticket a victory over Clinton-Kaine.

Cedar County's historic tie sixteen years earlier in 2000 reminded observers just how dynamic election results can be in a hear-'em-out agrarian region known for flipping its political allegiances with each election cycle, often voting for the man or woman instead of his or her party. But while the dead heat in my stomping grounds confirmed for me the validity of Woodard's map of rival regional cultures engaged in ideological tug-of-war, it also speaks to the geo-demographic differences that make the agrarian Midwest and Great Plains so politically precious. In his book *The Big Sort: Why the Clustering of Like-Minded America Is Tearing Us Apart* author Bill Bishop shares county-level presidential election results from Jimmy Carter vs. Gerald Ford in 1976 to Obama vs. McCain in 2008, mapping a partisan "big sort" across a thirty-two-year period during which, increasingly, American counties tipped to vote Republican or Democrat in landslides. In fact, between 1976 and 2004 only thirty-three percent of counties in American had grown more competitive, with the rest tipping dramatically into the Democratic or Republican column. The emerging majority of newly tipped counties dramatically decreased the number of purple places in which Americans live in close proximity to neighbors with political views dramatically different than their own.

The upshot? My purple city in my purple state in an increasingly purple home region—the Upper Midwest—now offers an increasingly rare privilege in America: the built-in civics lesson that comes with living in a truly diverse political ecology wherein geodemographically-diverse Democrats and Republicans roam the land in equal numbers. It turns out that agrarians who hang their hats in places like mine experience a political landscape of increasingly heirloom quality: not the bland orthodoxy of neighbors nodding their quiet Amens to every political protestation made at the local cafe, but free-thinking neighbors whose disparate votes suggest they will be equally inclined to disagree with us, respectfully.

Part V:

Seasons

Moving Beyond "It Could Have Been Worse"

In the nation's midsection spring means direct-line impacts from the sundry calamities our insurance agents put under the umbrella "Acts of God": tornadoes, floods, straight-line winds, hail sized pea- to baseball. In the wake of historic "bomb cyclones" and a barrage of spring storms national reporters descend to offer their sympathies while their cameras record ruined and washed-out lives. In their reports we emerge as an almost Biblical people, fated to endure drought and deluge and to bear up under it all, somehow, with a pioneer's faith and moxie we possessed long before their pressing deadlines.

For the record we do bear up, more often than not, and the otherwise well-intentioned members of the media assigned to report our cosmically bad luck jet back to LA or New York or Washington DC. Bags packed and news packages wrapped, they leave us to pick up the pieces. Contrary to the images they collect and curate we don't always look at the devastation God wrought and say in that John Wayne tone reserved for us in Hollywood movies, "Well, it could've been worse." Sometimes it's worse than we could ever have imagined. Sometimes, given space and trust, we're willing to say as much.

Sometimes we break down as soon as the cameras stop rolling. As a people we're humble enough to understand that every country must have its midlanders, a good and stalwart people whose collective hardships are regarded by the rest of a nation as a measuring stick for God's wrath and vengeance. Nature ensures the ultimate irony: that a place subject to the extremes of midcontinental weather must be populated by a people conditioned to prefer the middle in most things.

We're given to understand that every nation has its storm-prone places, as does every state and every city: postal codes where the catastrophic walls of water and damaging winds strike with disproportionate frequency and fury. Often the afflicted places are poor, illustrating the ugly truth of environmental gentrification and explaining why victims are more likely to be impoverished than those watching the calamities unfold on TV at a safe remove.

The drama of our severe weather hits us doubly each spring. Not only does it leave many of our struggling rural communities hurting, but it takes attention away from the other good and worthy things coming to bloom in the forgotten middle of the country: "Brain Gain" in some of our better-endowed rural counties, a record number of new "farms" (though far too many of them hobby and boutique), the blessing of our uniquely grassroots politics and historically tight-knit communities.

It's worth recalling each April and May, as the media zoom in on what's left of our lives scattered across the lawn like so many pick-up sticks, that we are more than the sum of our natural disasters, more than the projection of our collective grief at the magnitude of events beyond our control.

What we are is a stick-with-it people who want more than breezy and passing coverage.

New Diluvial Normal

Great Plains tornadoes are said to be strong enough to drive pieces of hay into fence posts, but the catastrophic floods that perennially impact my rural town of four hundred are just as capable of rearranging the status quo into surreal tableaus. Of the top ten historic crests recorded by the National Weather Service on my home river all have come during the last ten years, with the exception of the crest of 22.0 feet in 1968—the year my father graduated high school.

Though the rest of the country sees us as dish-pan flat and consequently uneventful, Middle America is a place of rivers, creeks, and wetlands. *Land-locked* does not adequately convey the depth and power of the roiling currents around us. While nearly 40 percent of the rest of the nation lives in counties boasting shoreline, midlanders live near the less heralded creeks, streams, ditches, and canals that drain our watersheds into the mid-sized rivers that, in turn, flow into the muddy Mississippi or Missouri Rivers, and south to the Gulf of Mexico.

Several years ago local news coverage of our particularly calamitous flood events led with the sanguine headline "Flood Victims…Depend on Themselves for Flood Protection." It's a sort of non-headline, actually, boiling down to the self-evident—rural people left to care for themselves. The reportage acknowledged that we have dealt with flooding almost every other year for the past ten years, and the journalist dispatched to detail our misfortune reported back, "Homeowners say they don't have city resources or volunteers to help protect them from flooding. Unlike in larger cities people [here] say they can only depend on themselves and their neighbors for protection." Still, while grim necessity makes us experts in helping one another through each successive deluge, we fail to help others understand how disproportionately we suffer from the new diluvial normal.

The Midwest is shaped by watersheds. The Missouri River, the longest in North America, drains more than half a million square miles, including ten states and two Canadian provinces. As our miles of paved roads and parking lots expand exponentially with regional urban development, and as the farming of what remains of our agricultural land grows more intense, the pressure on our waterways deepens as agricultural run-off increases. The acres of concrete and street level-drainage that coincide with the "smart growth" of the fastest growing regional cities (places like Columbus, Minneapolis, Indianapolis, and Grand Rapids) shunt floodwaters and run-off into our overburdened streams and drainage ditches. Like energy, water must go somewhere.

Every few years my town's city park and legion hall disappear beneath the roiling waters of the mostly undammed river in floods well-fed by the myriad waterways and arteries, named and unnamed, that drain our Grant Wood hills. And yet for all their frequency our river floods only become news when they affect our larger cities upstream, places big enough to evacuate apartment buildings in what makes for impressive news footage. Our plight and predicament reminds of the old Zen koan: if a tree falls in the woods and no one is there to hear it, does it make a sound?

If a tornado tears the roof off a barn or two somewhere in the Great Plains and never gets reported, in the eyes of metropolitan America, did it ever really happen?

Unlike a tornado, whose average ground speeds top thirty miles per hour, a flood, once begun, is inexorable and mostly predictable; its track is known in advance; its speed rarely exceeds six or seven miles per hour. By analogy a flood is more like a siege than a skirmish—a war of attrition lasting weeks rather than days. The headlines it generates reinforce a certain kind of monotony marked by the matter-of-fact reporting of record crests as they move downriver. An inundation is lived with; once precipitated, it carries little of the novelty news requires. Like Ben Franklin's quip about guests and fish, news of localized and regional flooding grows stale after a few days.

And unlike the major Midwestern cities whose downtown areas have been struck by EF1 and greater tornadoes in the last dozen years—places like Springfield, Missouri, and Des Moines and Iowa City, Iowa—a flood presents reporters with a moving target, demanding they follow it at some considerable inconvenience to their workaday lives. While the average tornado is on the ground for only five minutes, a river flood churns and roils its way forward for weeks, creating untold devastation.

Our new diluvial normal replenishes the wellspring of our original fatalistic thinking, the intrinsic understanding that all good things must end or change. Forests, farms, factories, family legacies—those best-laid plans of mice and men—are easily swept away in the end.

Summer Whirls

Summer is the perfect time to go antiquing. There's something deeply restorative about ducking into a dimly lit antique store on a midwestern Main when everyone and everything else has begun to wilt—like escaping into cathedral on a scorching summer day in Madrid or Milan to find a slip of peace far away from the bustling crowds.

Seldom these days do I enter a curio shop at home in small-town America without encountering a brood of orphaned globes huddled in some dusty corner. Whatever deficiencies caused their abandonment seem minor in retrospect. In some a once deep-blue Atlantic is faded to an off-hue; in others the Himalayan peaks have been rubbed flat by overzealous hands. Otherwise these tiny universes appear good as new.

Globes, those fixtures of Boomer and Gen X childhoods, are now the stuff of thrift-store clearance shelves. Plausible reasons abound—online maps, cheap, mass-market atlases beckoning beside the latest issue of *Cosmo* at nearly every check-out aisle—but the pleasures of a real globe are not easily replicated in two dimensions.

A real globe can be held in your hands, whirled to your heart's content, North America becoming a colorful blur. Back in the salad days before a real hole opened in the polar ozone, the globe at my grandparents' farmhouse was so well loved it developed a great gaping hole where the North Pole should have been, and wobbled worryingly on its axis when we passing grandkids gave it a breezy Harlem Globetrotters-styled spin.

Symbolically, the shunning of globes says something important about our culture. While we pay tribute in buzzwords like *global terror* and *global economy*, our notion of what *global* truly means grows more and more abstract. According to a Roper poll conducted for *National Geographic*, six out of ten 18- to 24-year-olds rumored to live in a "global culture" were unable to locate Iraq on a map of the Middle East. One-third couldn't find Louisiana post-Hurricane Katrina.

As dumb an instrument as a globe now seems to digital-age America, it offered a hands-on democratic education perfect for country kiddos. It didn't have to be dialed in or booted up or even turned on. In my childhood kids couldn't avoid globes, try as we might. So while my generation of rowdies broke them off their pedestals and used them as kickballs and basketballs, we were at least actively learning. To shoot a free throw with a globe liberated from its base was to know that the United States and Russia were indeed half a world apart. To palm a Rand McNally as if it were a Spalding basketball was to realize the immensity of the former Soviet Union, its eleven time zones exceeding the span of any outstretched kid-hand.

To touch a globe was instantly to know something about topography, geology, and natural history. Since the majority of the Midwestern and Great Plains states were pancake-flat under-finger, it stood to reason they were good for farming, especially the lush green Middle Western states, where the water flowed in blue-green veins toward the Mississippi. The Rockies, by contrast, were rough to the touch, a semi-arid inhospitable brown—in sum, a tough place to sink a plow; South Carolina and the coastal southeast were emphatically "Low Country." To own a globe was to put the United States in context, too—to realize we weren't quite as big as we thought we were, or to reconnoiter, with a gasp, that Cuba *was* only seventy miles from Key West.

To own a globe was to comprehend global change in practice. I grew up with a globe that didn't yet show breakaway Soviet republics like Lithuania, Chechnya, and the Ukraine, and yet that globe still serves despite featuring nonexistent countries such as Zaire (now the Democratic Republic of Congo) and Upper Volta, which up and changed its name to Burkina Faso "Land of upright men."

To keep or to buy a globe, no matter how old, is the equivalent of savoring an old address book that has grown gloriously out of date but which nevertheless stands for a lifetime of connections made and sometimes broken. To steal away on a summer's afternoon and take a globe for a spin is to acknowledge that both life and nation-building are dynamically unpredictable processes. To hold your own universe in your hands serves as a useful agrarian reminder that today's top dog may become tomorrow's bottom dweller.

Barefoot Eras

For a country kid barefooting represents a red badge of courage, a flaunting of the sage parental advice that warns children away from the plethora of small sharp objects planted beneath their tender feet—glass, nails, nettles, needles and beetles. You name it, it lurks beneath.

As kids my cousins and I viewed it as something more than a coincidence that the toughest among us, our cousin Leah, had feet as thick as horsehide and calluses deeper than any barnyard cowboy's. Leah, who rough-housed with the boys, was always first to dash across the rocky drive. While the rest of us winced and hollered and whooped and soft-shoed our way across—*eeh-ooh-ah*—as if stepping on hot coals, Leah practically levitated. She must have taken after my shoeless grandmother on my father's side who somehow managed to rule the roost without the usual dictator's props: iron fist and steel-toed boot. Half the time our empress wore no shoes.

Sometime between my grandmother's hog-calling, cow-rustling, bare-footed, pre-Depression-era youth and my own Generation X pussyfooting, barefooting became verboten. "Barefoot and pregnant" became the worst insult you could hurl a young woman's way, as if the two separate slurs—"barefoot" and "pregnant"—shared some sinister root. In my childhood signs suddenly went up on Main declaring, "No shirt, No shoes.

No service." The women in my family hemmed and hawed at the new-fangled prohibition, but ultimately they did as women so often do—adapted. My mom carried a pair of clogs, while my grandma toted her flip-flops—what she called her "clippees" for the *clip-clip* sound they produced whenever rubber sole smacked under-ankle. This "emergency" footwear hung out in the car in the event commerce needed doing—the way the men in our family carried tire irons and jumper cables.

As we kids watched and waited in the car, our heroine du jour would emerge triumphant from the dime store, twirling her shopping bags, looking like a million bucks. Then the car door would swing open on its rusty hinges and our ladies of perpetual subterfuge would kick off those insufferable shoes, put their big, bunyuned toes on the accelerator, and push the pedal to the metal, flooring it out of town. None of us took much truck from the foot police.

It's possible, I think, to grab hold of the decades by their shoestrings. The free-spirited Seventies can be understood as flip-flops and bell bottoms; the business-like Eighties are so much patent leather and pumps; the dawn-of-the-digital-age Nineties are pumped-up space-age high-tops, and so on.

Now it's the true barefooters among us—the real, raw dogs—that are threatened with extinction amid record sales for insoles, orthopedics, flip-flops, and sandals. Gone are the employees who used to "air out" beneath their desks, kicking off both shoes and socks. Gone are the days when going bootless meant not having to worry about the indignities of Chinese-made sweatshop sneakers. Gone, too, are the tough kids like Leah who could run a rock gauntlet in no time flat.

Still, we can take comfort in this bit of sole: today's kids are finding their feet again. Flip-flops are once more the rage even though kids today don't wear them like we used to—as a bit of practical passive cooling in the days before widespread A.C. Now they're donned as a fashion statement, an emblem of some wished for leisure, or else a retro homage to a past that seems more carefree when viewed in hindsight.

And the next generation seems to have what we lacked—the chutzpah to wear "clippees" to class and clogs to church. Can the risks inherent in daring to be barefoot and beautiful be far behind?

Then as now being yourself, consequences be damned, is no small feat.

Skunk Hours

Wildlife biologists are fond of pointing out that the skunk and man meet-up is one of the most frequent of all animal-human encounters. But when once my family hurried home through heavy summer air rife with "ode de skunk"; when once a dead skunk in the middle of the road became a national cliché and a hit song of the same name for folk singer Loudon Wainwright III, the skunk has left the scene without a scent.

If you'd rather not follow your nose to confirm the disappearance, you need only follow the road. Roadkill counts in 1980 taken by the Illinois Department of Natural Resources documented 2,618 dead skunks, or 4.83 per thousand road miles. Twenty-odd years later, the *Chicago Sun-Times* reported only 590 of the stinkers, or about .97 per thousand road miles. It's a macabre culture that keeps its finger on the pulse of its wildlife by counting the deceased. Still, you've got to hand it to the roadside morticians: their body count offers concrete evidence of a decline otherwise hard to measure in a population of known night owls.

The loss of skunks and all the odiferous memories that go with them constitute a national trend. Experts nationwide conduct necropsies to determine the source of the decimation, but so far the verdict remains out. Theories range from competition with well-fed raccoons to tick-borne illnesses. And while it's surely nothing more than odd coincidence or half-baked conspiracy theory, it's worth noting that during the same period that skunk litters have decreased by half, sales of air fresheners to U.S. households have gone through the roof, up nearly 30 percent.

Beyond the amorous Looney Tunes antics of Pepe Le Peu, the skunk captures a child's imagination as few animals do. Natural bedfellows, skunks and children have a strong affinity for one another, both being smelly and underfoot at the least opportune times. Skunks have always been a vital totem for kids who felt slighted, unwelcome, or otherwise verboten. Moreover, without frequent skunk encounters today's kids miss the mystical deskunkification defunking rites of a rural or small-town childhood, foremost among them the dunking of the family pet in tomato juice to remove the skunk's glandular stench.

Tradition in my farm family held that the first person to smell a skunk as we drove through its airborne essence had to say "I ONE it"; the second person "I TWO it" and so on around our old blue Pontiac until the unfortunate soul who had to say "I EIGHT (ate) it." It was a homespun agrarian version of Slug Bug—something to pass the time back in those long-ago summer-sweet days when chances of smelling a skunk equaled or rivaled those of spotting a Volkswagen Bug.

Seasonal Disaffections

January is more difficult to bear for rural and small-town residents. That sounds like the world's smallest violin playing its woeful tune, but it's true. Just ask any of the many resident rural grumps who develop a chip on their shoulder circa the first of the year and keep it there until the last of the ice melts.

We are, after all, an outdoor people relative to the rest of Pencil-Pusher Nation. When winter plays hardball it means we're mostly displaced not just from a workplace—often a farm, field, or feedlot—but from the heart and soul of a fresh-air profession, and therefore, an identity. An urban American might call the sudden weather-related loss of one's very job a bona fide existential crisis. Here we just cuss it out and call it winter.

Sure, work gets done on the farm or ranch regardless of how far the mercury drops, but what bites most about a country winter is the sting inherent in the loss of control it brings. We are a thoroughly controlling people, most of us rural routers are—well-nigh impossible to please, intolerant of incompetence, possessed of Type A personalities that work famously well in the stockyards and barnyards but don't exactly fly these days in the touchy-feely markets of Match.com or eHarmony.

We're skilled controllers not just because some Alpha-Controller in our family once painstakingly showed us how from step A to step Z, but because we have to be. Everything must get done right and right now, or Mother Nature ensures there will be hell to pay. Choose the easy chair in lieu of the snow blade on the day after the latest in a perverse season's parade of storms, and an obliging arctic cold front blows in and freezes the snowdrifts you left in the lane solid until St. Patty's Day. The indignity of the permanently drifted-in-drive, in turn, means the cold shoulder of the Better Half, and ushers in a season of frigid weather and a bed whose sudden chill has more to do with disappointed expectations than bitter north winds. How many kindly and enlightened country spouses and partners, helpless before the grim seasonal disaffections that descend on their loved ones like low pressure systems, have appealed in earnest to the angels of their mate's better nature, saying of this ill-intentioned season, "But, honey, there's nothing you can do about it." Of course, the nothing-to-do-about-it is exactly the crux of the problem.

Especially in the dark days of winter, minutes matter, machinery matters, and method matters, all of which stoke the fire of the perennial perfectionist. Ask any stockman or woman and they'll tell you control in a month like January isn't merely a matter of style; it's a matter of survival. Of course the farmer and the rancher would live longer and at a substantially lower blood pressure if they would only make their peace with the ultimate cage-rattler: Old Man Winter. But to call a truce with such a prodigious bully would be to run contrary to exactly the fighting spirit that allowed their kin to settle such chilly climes in the first place.

To do as all the citified psychotherapists and New Agers would have us do—*take a deep breath, detach, accept, go-with-the-flow*—doesn't stick with us for the same reason we persist in eating buttermilk biscuits and breaded tenderloins the size of dinner plates—because being who we always have been, which is to say true to ourselves, is something valued here where change is designed to be hard to come by. It's our very predictability that differentiates us from our cousins in the city, who not only seek change but invite it in and pour it a hot toddy.

Many of us learned our controlling ways from our farming grandmas and grandpas, and along with it the certain knowledge that when you stop fighting and surrender to winter in favor of the easy chair and daytime television, you're as good as dead anyway. Show me a rural dweller living north of Nashville, Tennessee, who really and truly relishes winter, and I'll show you either a native Minnesotan, Michigander, or someone who drew a regular paycheck in town their entire working life and who's quietly incubating through this leanest of seasons a particularly fat pension or an especially robust nest egg.

They're easy enough to ferret out in the wintry countryside, these crowing winter boosters. They're given away by the light in their eye when they answer the door cheerily on a morning when it's twenty below zero, by the way they pull their comb through their coiffed yet slightly mussed hair before joining you outside for a chit-chat beside their rust-free, all-wheel-drive Acura parked in the drive. When they start proselytizing on the pleasures of snow-shoeing and cross-country skiing and all the other positively delightful winter sports practically no one subscribes to in these parts, it's better just to politely lower your head and stare at your boots till their well-meaning sermon is over. Odds are these chirpy advocates of winter have two tickets to Orlando warming in their thermals. And it's true: winter might be tolerable if you had a way to escape it, or if you hadn't battled it like a barroom brawler from the time you were old enough to drive a tractor.

Me, I learned seasonal disaffections under the tutelage of a master—my farming grandfather—who from Easter to Thanksgiving was as lovely and gentle a shepherd as ever trod the greening pastures, but who became the biggest bad-weather bear you ever saw at first snowfall. As a teenager I found endless amusement in his dark seasonal grumblings—that is, until I grew up and began plowing out my own rural route. Then, and without even thinking, I reached back to borrow my winter color-scheme from him—a veritable palette of grays and blues.

Winter's most redeeming truth lies in such cold and unerring symmetries.

Mind of Winter

The poet Wallace Stevens wrote about something he called the "Mind of Winter." But for an agrarian like me winter begins at the feet.

Numb feet serve as a natural governor of my Protestant work ethic and my tendency to "overdo it," as my father (a farmer-overdoer if ever there was one) always said. He also said, "You don't need to shoot yourself in the foot to know that it hurts," another one-size-fits-all, podiatrical metaphor perfectly apt for overzealousness on the farm or off it.

When I was a boy we never thought to name winter storms for breezy rogues or cold jezebels. Instead of arriving at our door sporting names like Octavia, Hektor, and Pandora, our storms came bearing more homely monikers: Looks Real Bad, or my grandfather's favorite, Damn It All to Hell. Back then no glad-handing, good Sam of a citified, certified weatherman had to tell us to stay home when the weather soured and the winds turned wicked. Staying home was precisely what the spade-work of planting and sowing and digging out entailed. In ordinary weather the prospect of going to town positively underwhelmed. The thought of going there when the North winds howled and a Hektor or a Wolf or a Gorgon had us by the shorthairs had us doubly nonplussed.

I appreciate now the subtle ways winter brought us together. It brought my father and grandfather down from the Olympian heights of their John Deere cabs to do something plain and plebian like shovel snow with women and children. Snow-moving and other winter sports on the farm fell into predictable patterns once the hard-driven men blew in. First, we would work on the hairy, maniacal edge of frostbite for what seemed like days until someone in the group, usually an elder, would lean on their shovel and declare "Whaddya say we go in and warm up for a spell?" What they really meant was "Jesus, I can't feel my toes!" or "Mary Mother of God, we've got to get inside before we all perish!" but they couldn't let on. It's fair to say that during the other nine months of the year I believed my farm elders were invincible. I never once heard them say the word "can't," for example. Never did I hear them utter, "Shoot, we might as well just throw in the towel and watch us some cable."

Still winter and its chill gave them proper pause. Retreating into the house for a brief warm-up didn't constitute defeat. We had merely retired to rally the troops and stoke our flagging fires. Coffee and hot cocoa and a fresh pair of wool socks were our way of saying, Look out, you son-of-a-bitch-of-the-mother-of-all-winter-storms, we're coming for you when we're good and ready.

Many years have passed since the first time I saw Old Man Winter turn my family's otherwise invincible elders back inside with us kids in tow. Nowadays, when I hear my farm scoopmate or shovel-buddy mouth the sweet words, "Let's go in and warm up a bit," I think about grace—how it never falls out of fashion, how stopping to warm up is nothing more nor less than a timely acknowledgement of human limits. And when I think back on recent years of political gridlock, pandemic, and rampant and ruthless war, I think there must be something truly wise in leaning on one's shovel to propose not a capitulation but a temporary cessation. There must be something holy in coming in to regroup at the exact moment when the feet begin to tingle, the heart begins to fail, and the body can no longer bear what the eye despairs.

Today, tomorrow, or ten minutes from now, mountains will still need moving. And if we intend to be standing when heaven and earth are moved, we'll want to be able to feel our toes.

February's Got Teeth

In a world of few absolutes it's fair to say that practically no one likes to lie down for the dentist, and that's especially true, I'd argue, for rural folks. It's a bona fide aversion, deep as an abscess, and it's worth rooting out how it came to be.

February, as irony has it, is National Dental Health Month. The timing makes a perverse kind of sense in a family like mine, where Dr. Drill finishes a close second to Old Man Winter in our perennial unpopularity contest. I myself come from an exceptionally fine pedigree of dental health skeptics and conspiracy theorists, including a grandmother who practiced expert avoidance until her late eighties, when the four grown children she had labored to bring into the world, kicking and screaming, forced her, kicking and screaming, into a complete set of dentures. My own dental-avoidance stats pale in comparison to Gran's, though they proudly topped ten years until recently, when, rotten as the proverbial apple, a molar in the way-back of my mouth fell out into my soup bowl, and I was forced to go in for a check-up.

It's not every day a body part falls into your lap or your homemade chili. And when it does it's bound to yield several days of existential soul-searching, beginning with: why is the janitorial staff tasked with the upkeep of my so-called bodily temple falling down on the job so much lately?

Then comes the self-incriminating self-talk: "I really should take better care of myself," we conscientious agrarians lecture ourselves. After the prosecution rests things really start to get interesting. It's at this point we begin to ask whether we needed the damn thing in the first place, and commence to prying and probing around in our mouth like we would in the crankcase of a combine—shining a trouble light here, tapping with a ball-peen there—cautiously opening it up to see if she'll still run despite the bad or missing parts. What is a tooth, anyhow, but a fragment of a broken flywheel?

The next step in the dental recovery process is the most thoroughly countrified—in other words no twelve-step Kubler-Ross psycho-babble need apply. I call this step the Invention Phase, and it's basically this: something is broken; that something will cost thousands of dollars and loads of time to haul into town to have somebody in a uniform take a look at it, sigh deeply, and slide a bill across the desk with a multi-step treatment plan that'll cost us as much as a zero turn-radius mower with all the bells and whistles. If there's one thing we rural denizens pride ourselves in doing without, it's the so-called expert in town with his credentials framed on the wall and pile of glib glossy magazines on the table that no one around here subscribes to anyhow.

Taken on its own terms rural repurposing is a glorious thing, demonstrating not just the ingenuity of our people but our perfectly legitimate tradition of doing by and for ourselves. On the farm or ranch there's always something around that looks and acts akin to the thing that's gone missing, and that's where the fun comes in. That's when the scrap pile behind the barn or the junk drawer in the service shed is as good as any overpriced parts department and way better than an overcrowded waiting room.

I for one never feel more whole than when I'm taking a broken thing and putting it back together again, on the fly, with what's left of the good sense I was born with. I'm sure all the soft-voiced psychotherapists in town would have a field day with such a revelation, but for me, not having to drive to the city to buy the gee-whiz part, even when that part might be a color-matched tooth filling, is an unqualified victory...a score for rurality. Granted, Extreme DIY of the kind I sometimes malpractice is its own pathology, as anyone will tell you who's had a badly jerry-rigged Band-Aid cure quite literally blow up in their face. Indeed, some of my own barnyard workarounds best belong in the category of Hall of Shame or World's Worst Fixes, including anything I've ever tried to solder and the expired rubber cement I recently tried in lieu of plumber's adhesive. All of which brings me full circle to the missing tooth and my recent, wholly involuntary trip to the dentist. The highly credentialed expert behind the drill informed me with a cosmetically-correct grin that my ten years of ignorance-is-bliss was now going to cost me as much as a brand new car.

Even if I did have the dead presidents to roto-rooter out the dead roots and build up the missing tooth myself, I intend to do no such thing, at least not anytime soon. So long as I'm paying out of pocket I'm thinking of what I might use instead to whip up a barnyard denture...some Bondo maybe or a fiberglass repair kit. Or how about that old country standby: wood, freshly primed and enameled? If it was good enough for gentleman farmer

George Washington when the old chompers broke down in the field, then it's good enough for me.

And what about the rotten old tooth, the one that kamikazed into my bowl of chili? I'm thinking it might make a capital game piece for the next time I'm forced to drive my toothless self into town to play Oral Health Care Monopoly—the game we keep playing even when we're bound to end up bankrupt.

Time for Cheering

Had my mother not been a cheerleader for our hometown Mustangs and a winsome waitress at the local A & W drive-in, chances are good I wouldn't be here and neither would many of my Gen X brethren. My father won't say whether it was the ice cream she carried on summer weekends or the poms she sported on game nights that sealed the deal, but I imagine her cheerleader status didn't hurt.

Before today's holier-than-thou, politically-correct readers look askance at the "shimmy up a toothpick, slide down a straw" cheerleaders who take the field each August let me hasten to add that we lose more than we think when old-fashioned cheerleaders hang up the poms.

In my mid-twenties I took a job as a small-town newspaper section editor not far from our family's Heritage Farm. I set up shop in the first few weeks of December when the snow was still fresh and the spirits high. I spent the better part of a month covering basketball in stuffy gymnasiums before I correctly attributed the hush that had settled over the proceedings to the absence of cheerleaders.

Ever the cub reporter, I asked around until I learned that cheerleading in small towns had slipped a rung or two on the coolness ladder. There hadn't been enough interest that winter to field a squad. While sucking on a Twizzler rope one night at halftime, a high school teacher kindly explained to me that today's kids want to play sports, not merely cheer for them.

It's wonderful that we as a culture want to be in the game, and yet pretending as if being in the game is the only thing that matters inevitably leads to the disparagement of the cheerleading spirit. Sadly, it's become uncool to cheerlead, in a literal as well as a figurative sense. By comparison it's hyper fashionable to be a "whistleblower" so much that a simple web search for the aforementioned results in some three million hits over just a three-month time period. During the same timeframe use of *whistleblower* relative to *cheerleader* has grown exponentially. It seems it's sexier now to tattle tale, kiss and tell, or simply rat out those in the spotlight than to make nice from the sidelines. Better to be a disgruntled, often complicit, participant-critic-snitch, the whistleblower versus cheerleader dichotomy seems to say, than a mere bystander, no matter how cheerful.

In the current cultural moment, cheerleading, like so many homegrown products turned exports, is now deemed distasteful, decadent, or simply déclassé by many Americans. Overseas it's another story entirely. A recent *Newsweek* story headlined its coverage of the Cheerleading Worlds competition—described as "the Super Bowl of spirit competitions"—by detailing the unlikely successes of China's Nanning Middle School No. 26 squad. The ever-industrious Chinese, writes Arian Camp Flores, have figured out that "cheer's camaraderie will fight the isolation many of China's studious children feel and ever since they've been investing in it, and investing heavily."

It's not that cheerleading has become passé in the U.S.A., but that what passes as cheering today is qualitatively different in spirit than the cheerleading most of us remember. Back then it wasn't a stand-alone sport but a vital and symbiotic accompaniment, no more and no less than the band. To discount the kind of traditional sideline cheerleading of yore is something akin to declaring the drum corps worthless to Civil War soldiers or the boogie-woogie buglers incidental to American doughboys.

Fifteen-year-old sprite Nicole Pelillo typifies the needs of the new-fangled cheerleader. Pelillo is quoted in a recent *Time* magazine saying that she hates "sideline cheering" because the fans packing the stands cheer for the football team, not for her.

While cheerleaders and cheerleading survive in name, the purer virtues of cheerleading of the kind our grandparents practiced when they dropped everything in order to root us on from the stands now find themselves at the bottom of the pyramid. Gran and Gramps didn't cheer us on from the bench because they wanted the spotlight to be on them. They didn't attend as disgruntled would-be participants, hungry for attention and upset if they didn't get it. They were there to be a support, to focus attention on us in order to will us, by dint of their concentration, to better and better-spirited play.

As their cheerful devotion proved, a little sis-boom-bah never falls out of fashion.

Twilight-time: An Open Letter

Twilight tonight couldn't make up its mind. Last weekend Gran called it messy, and she sat there, ninety-years-old in May, looking very satisfied with it, I guess because life is beautiful in a messy way.

Graduation is this Saturday and then I start teaching summer school, but don't feel sorry for me. Just one class and quite a bit more time knocking around home. I like how the hours swell in the summer, and I like days when the biggest decision is what to have for dessert: popsicle or ice cream. Lately, it's ice cream, hands down, sometimes out of a measuring cup, when the bowls get used up; other times straight out of the carton like a raccoon.

Each day I take a different cardinal direction on my walk, though I never seem to go North, I guess because in the old maps the wind blows from up there, all icy and full of himself. If I have my druthers I'll follow the sloughs south. Sometimes I stay on the blacktop going straight toward the river, but if it's too hot I cross over onto the gravel road. I like that way because it's flat until the bridge, which is a good place to pause, pat yourself on the back for coming this far, and think cool watery thoughts. Then it's straight uphill if you want to earn the view of town where the schoolhouse looks storybook.

On my way back this time a red-winged blackbird put me in its crosshairs and wouldn't let go, screeching as if I had stolen its first-born. Face to face a scorned red-wing looks like an angry headmaster and sounds like a sharp-tongued county clerk. But then they're scarier than that, too, those red-wings, and I don't suppose there's anything human to which to compare them.

After a half mile or so of craning to see my attacker, my neck started hurting, so I kept track of the red-wing's antics by following its shadow on the rock roadbed, like a vulture's cast onto a canyon floor. The bird-shadow looked like Batman for a bit, then like the angel of death. This bright, beautiful day and this dark, dark bird with flames for wings and that gravel road always like an afterlife—flat, flat, flat and the crest of the hill close but never getting any closer. What is it the Irish say in their blessing…may the road rise to meet you?

I'm still halfway looking for a new house. Sometimes I worry I'm too weary for the rigmarole of a new place…all the newness, which I guess is what stops widows. It seems like no matter whom you're mortgaged to you always end up calling some bright-eyed, bushy-tailed, twenty-something in Des Moines who is all too glad to arrange for payment. I always wonder how they can stay so happy there in their cubicles. Probably it's the kind of happiness that comes when someone else is paying for the air-conditioning.

Homes on paved roads fetch higher resale prices, it's true, but I like dusty rural routes like the one I grew up on. Say what you will about gravel chewing up Goodyears and chipping clear coats, but it's a great way to keep the crowd from your door even if your ditch lilies do get dusty. You can choose a husband or wife that way, too, by taking your forefinger and seeing how much dust is on them, like they do with coffee tables in furniture polish commercials. Usually the dustier the better.

Gravel roads remind of how Grampy used to pick up rocks down on his hands and knees in the ditch, nit-picking. Seeing a farmer on his knees never did sit right with me. If you were picking up rocks with Grampy, you had to be sure to pick up anything bigger than a pea. With Dad, it was anything bigger than a marble, and by the time you're helping me pick rocks out of my ditch, I'll bring my forefinger and thumb together to make the universal symbol for "Leave it, it's smaller than a quarter." Then we'll call it a day and have some ice cream. Ice cream breaks at midday…that's what the curmudgeons mean when they say the younger generation is going to hell in a handbasket.

I started my bike ride too late tonight and didn't get in until dark. I didn't meet too many cars on the road, thank goodness, but I did meet one of those huge "high-boy" boom sprayers, the ones that look like giant grasshoppers with their wings tucked back in attack mode. It was road-hogging. I couldn't see the man behind the machine, but I could see the sunset smeared all over his plate glass window.

I should probably pause here to communicate a few things of deep and abiding importance to me, things like cherish your heritage, sink deep roots, and live without fear. But what I really want to say is this: when I saw that big boom sprayer barreling down the road I wanted to ride right under him, like you see in the action movies where a semi truck is gunning for the hero and there's no way out until our hero lays flat on the ground and the truck passes right over them. Straight into the belly of the whale, I say.

So there you have it—the larger life lesson you and I would just as soon avoid speaking for fear of sounding preachy, or weepy, or just plain precious.

Always, always do your own stunts.

Rural Rip Van Winkle

Twenty years ago I was a twenty-something occasional poet and journalist looking for a good university at which to pursue my passion for writing. I had spent years sinking meaningful roots in my local farm community, occupying positions like small-town library clerk and newspaper section editor that brought me intimately close to my neighbors and our shared place.

But the youthful part of me still yearned for adventure. So when a former professor of mine told me I should give New Mexico a try I listened. She had recently returned from a visiting professorship there, and said she had never seen a place so diverse—hippies, commies, Native Americans, environmentalists, ranchers, foodies, and survivalists somehow living side by side. You name it, she said, and New Mexico had it with a side of chiles.

And the rest, as they say, is history. Except that it isn't, not purely.

I left Las Cruces, New Mexico, an aspiring writer and return now as an author, but that's not what's so poignant about coming back, or so scary. Like many writers I've been better at reimagining others' pasts then at revisiting my own. When Facebook first hit the scene, for example, friends of mine reported breathless online encounters with friends and frenemies from decades ago. Hearing the giddy stories of their personal exhumations only reinforced in me a decided need to live in the present. I had stayed in contact with my best friends from long ago, I told them, and if I hadn't, then maybe they were destined to remain ghosts of the past.

Now, somewhere north of 40 (the age rather than the Interstate), I see that the ghosts return whether you will or you won't, and that circles, rather than straight lines, describe how life moves, drawing us back in concentric loops while at the same time spinning us forward, further down the road, into the unknown. Life imitates literature that way: like a good whodunit you finish a chapter only to find yourself circling back to suss out the small yet crucial details and divinities missed along the way.

Though it seems like the proverbial blink of an eye, twenty years is a full generation, and as I search online now for professors I had back then, I find that not a single one of them remains exactly where I left them; several have retired and became emeriti; others semi-retired and now teach online; others moved on to teach at other fine universities. One who was especially kind to me tragically took her own life.

Returning to a place you loved at a time when you loved life and all its vicissitudes is like the Heraclitean River; the river may be the same, but you who dip your toes in it have changed, and therefore you can never step into the same river twice. And even if you could revisit the places of your past perfectly preserved, as exactly the same person you were back then, would you want to?

For me Las Cruces, New Mexico, even beyond the time I spent there at the university, was a teacher; it taught me that rich didn't necessarily mean happy; that it was possible for a dizzying variety of divergent people to productively share the same beautiful valley in addition to other lessons big and small. The ruins of the old tuberculosis sanatoriums in the foothills taught me that the desert was once a place to which Americans escaped en masse to heal, and that it will be so again; history, Mark Twain once said, doesn't exactly repeat itself, but it does rhyme.

Everywhere in this most agrarian of valleys I found lessons waiting to be reaped. The haunty, flooded-by-design pecan fields of old Mesilla, where the youthful Billy the Kidd once romped and roamed, reminded me that every sentient, living thing should be capable of turning sudden surplus into sustenance, deluge into daily bread. The late summer chile harvest in Hatch served as a living reminder not to jump the gun, that the merciless desert heat and sun of June and July added character and flavor, that good things were worth waiting for.

The switchback trails over the Organ Mountains taught me that it was sometimes a good idea to let others know where you were going, and to be mindful of scorpions en route; a greasy-spoon desert café called the Golden Bull taught me that it's good to be the kind of person who stays long enough in one place to find your coffee cup still hanging on its hook when you return. The desert in springtime taught me to hang on, that the winds play devil; the wet season, when it arrived, showed me that students in the Southwest sometimes need to take "rain days" the way Midwesterners take snow days. The snow on the mountains, when it stuck, taught me that every place has a winter, and that every season, in a place as in a life, has a beauty all its own.

Agrarian and rural places often push young (and younger) men away from circumspection into head-down, get 'er done unsentimentalism. Remembrance, memorialization, open nostalgia… all these we tolerate (and sometimes celebrate) in men nearing old age or retirement, while simultaneously refusing or denying them to our young guns and warriors lest they threaten to unman them.

I for one am grateful that I fell in love with a fertile desert valley many moons ago, and I am doubly grateful, twenty years later, for the good, hard work of closing up circles—of planting my feet there once again, if only for a season.

The river, I am glad to say, still runs.

Autumnal Swings

Tire swings are a remnant of a do-it-yourself agrarian age, a long-ago day when a farmer's wife might be overheard saying, "Now, John, you *will* let me know when you change the tires on the old truck, won't you? I want to set one aside for the kids." Such complex negotiations over shared resources required great marital patience and fortitude—a good example for little ears, in any case.

My aunt Nan had a tire swing, still does in fact, along with that perfect little patch of dust above which it comes to a pendulum's rest. There the self-swingers scrapped the ground to stop their swing, and there the "pushers" braced themselves to slow the swinger who screamed "Enough, "I want off," "That's too high!" or, worst of all, "I'm going to be sick!"

Of course a tire swing is a non-starter unless an unused radial can be found bouncing around the backyard somewhere, and that's increasingly rare. Few Americans care to change a tire for themselves anymore; still fewer know how. Statistics say that up to 92 percent of the driving public doesn't know how to fix a flat. These days, too, the spent rubbers the tire guys take off at the Jiffy Lube or the Goodyear end up in everything from high-tech running tracks to the soles of shoes. That's a good thing, but not if you're a tire swing or a tire-swinger.

Tires have been recycled around the farm and ranch since the dawn of the internal combustion engine—in my own farmyard I enlist two tractor tires to keep my day lilies in check—it's how and why we recycle them that's changed. Whereas a generation ago recycling amounted to a homespun imaginative act of redemption and repurposing, i.e., what could you do around the farmyard with that rusty old spaghetti strainer, it's now become, like most things in American life, a service others provide to save us the time and trouble. So while the feel-goods belong to us, the tire-recycling consumer, the labor, the profit, and the knowledge belong to someone else, usually the recycling company that picks up and carts away what we lack the imagination to reuse.

Naturally, the tire swing, like that other playground dinosaur, the monkey bars, is dangerous, as anyone knows who's been walloped blindside by a thirty-five pound Michelin with some serious Isaac Newtons behind it. Sure, the homely tire swing lacks the satisfying suburban control offered by the swing set, from whose soaring vantage point it seems possible to own the world. On a playground swing you pump your legs to precisely control your distance, arc, and speed. On a tire swing you simply hang on for dear life, while the rope above you twists like a pretzel, the tree limb groans under your weight, and your rope ultimately unwinds in a thousand nausea-inducing circles. That kind of just-like-life ride may not sound like much fun to the unlucky soul who's never tried, but it is, precisely because it is a challenge to get on and stay on.

Not too many great ideas, I imagine, have been born on a tire swing; not many moms and dads have had to call out, "You can play more on the tire swing tomorrow, it's time for dinner!"

But in the peculiarly sweet wounds it inflicted on generations of country kids, the much maligned, now mostly forgotten tire swing offered some irreplaceable life lessons, namely the fine line between pain and pleasure.

In one of his lesser-known take-it-easy summer anthems Jimmy Buffet compared life to a tire swing. And I think what he meant was that a ride on a tire swing is a lot like life: slow in the beginning, breathless in the middle, and bittersweet in the end.

Afterword: A Look Back at *Country Views*

Over the decade in which the columns and commentaries collected herein were written much has changed in the life of rural America. That life in the countryside has changed so much in such a relatively short time is itself a challenge to the agrarian mind, which, when forced to choose, often chooses to slow time rather than to hasten it, the breakneck pace of contemporary culture itself a dangerous headlong rush toward an uncertain outcome.

Shortly after the first of these commentaries was written my father passed away, leaving me to contemplate even more deeply our shared legacy on the land. In fact, it took me years of intense grieving, thinking, and difficult living to ready myself to write about his loss. My father's passing in early 2011 followed my grandfather's, grandmother's, and uncle's in relatively close succession, taking with them my most direct links to our historic profession: farming. In some important way each of the pieces collected in *Country Views* was born of that loss, for I was mourning not just the loss of the three most important people in my life, but also lamenting the passing of a way of life.

The absence of these guardian spirits proved galvanizing. Who was I now that they had gone? Who did I want to be? What remained to be pieced back together? On the other hand, what was left that should be burned, so that I might begin again, from ashes? What would become of the values they stood for? What would become of the land they reaped and sowed, cultivated and cared for? For more than three decades I had been an apprentice, an understudy, a bench-warmer. Now circumstance forced me out onto the field to play like my life depended on it, and in many ways it did.

As the bereaved in my family gradually moved from the farm back to town, I resolved to root down in the place where I was originally planted. Mine wasn't a simple decision—my livelihood required me to travel and to teach—but it was rooting by choice, and thus one of the first, most powerful choices a person can make of their own free will. At times I chastised myself for the headstrong nature of my choice, suspecting stubbornness and intractability where I preferred to see enlightenment. At other times I was proud of the way I had, to borrow one of my father's favorite sayings, "voted with my feet" for a life I admired but doubted whether I could still live. At weaker moments I worried I had become a case of arrested development.

One of the later commentaries collected here, "Our Ancestors Sleep Down the Road," was one of several that garnered an almost instantaneous response from readers when it appeared in the *Des Moines Register* in the late spring of 2016. It had taken me more than five years to come to terms with the loss of my forebears on the farm. Then one mild May afternoon, triggered by the impending Memorial Day holiday, the words came tumbling out. Only when I had finished getting them down on paper did I recognize on the page the first signs that I had begun to heal, to come to terms with the personal and cultural losses of a culture—agriculture—that constitutes our beating heart.

The voice that came out surprised me. Was I indignant and a bit angry at the fate that had befallen my father and many of his peers? I was. Was I lucky to count myself among the living and breathing, still with a voice, an axe to grind, and blessings and benedictions to share? I was.

I had asked myself who I was, and now, five years later, I had my answer in writing.

Increasingly my agrarian op-eds and commentaries drew reply from urban and suburban readers. The vast majority wrote in support, a few wrote in indignation, and one or two with something approaching envy for the bucolic life they imagined I must be leading. Sometimes indignation mingled curiously with envy in letters-to-the-editor written in response to my commentaries, replies like this one from Jane in Des Moines:

> I wonder if Zachary Michael Jack realizes how fortunate and privileged he is to have his ancestors sleeping just down the road from where he lives. Many of us do not share that luxury. I am one of those whom he chides for having an "urban" mindset. My ancestors are, unfortunately, scattered across this great country. The most recent grandmothers and great uncles live on in my memory. However, I believe I can be forgiven if I visit some of these ancestors only on Memorial Day since I must fly hundreds of miles to do so. So, enjoy your good fortune, Mr. Jack. Massachusetts is a long way from Iowa!

When readers like Jane published their rejoinders I knew I had touched a nerve, often, ironically, among people more like me than different, despite our superficial demographic differences. What did Jane, who lived in a capital city of nearly a quarter million, have in common with me, living on a farm outside of a town of 400 without so much as a stoplight? Jane cared enough about her community to read the newspaper, and when she found in its pages something that compelled her, she was moved to write. She honors her family's dead on Memorial Day. And she wishes she could be closer to them still, so that she might do an even better job. These attributes make the writer and the reader, even when seemingly on opposite sides of an issue, far more similar than dissimilar. He or she who moves us to deeper thinking even when they sometimes make us mad is in many ways our truest friend.

I understood the blessings of my singular life, but surely Jane could see, couldn't she, that to have so many family members pass away at such a relatively young age did not qualify me as lucky? My commentary had not been penned to boast of sleeping each night a quarter mile down the road from my ancestors, but as a way to find redemptive value in the personal tragedies that had so abundantly populated our family graveyard.

Exchanges like these proved to me that though I was by nature adverse to notoriety I was willing to serve as a lightning rod for the issues about which I cared mostly deeply, and willing to pay the price for publishing in the popular press impassioned pleas no less fierce in their advocacy for rural and small-town people than those city dwellers routinely placed in urban media.

Other commentaries and opinion pieces drew responses on and off the page as well, letting me know that the voice I had recovered with such difficulty was resonating. Shortly after "We're Dying Here" appeared in the *Daily Yonder* in 2014 I received an email from an economist in the United States Department of Agriculture. She wrote that my op-ed had caused her to propose that her agency conduct further research on the shocking disparities between rural and urban life expectancies. That piece, published in the chronological middle of the pieces collected in *Country Views*, reminded me that I wasn't just whistling in the graveyard, that there were others who shared my agrarian heart and mind, and who were likewise urgently looking for answers.

One of the more recent agrarian commentaries collected here, an op-ed from June 2017 entitled "We Live and Die by Chemical Agriculture" drew commentary from across the state and region, most in sympathy with its call for common-sense public protections against pesticide and herbicide drift. Robert wrote from Marshalltown, Iowa:

> Zachary Michael Jack wrote of Iowa's dependence on chemical agriculture [We live and die by chemical agriculture, June 9]. A point he neglects to make is that farmers are now working thousands of acres, rather than the hundreds of acres per farm back in the 1970s. In addition, fewer and fewer farmers do their own spraying because of equipment, hazards and time. Spraying is being done by co-ops spraying multi-thousand acres and they have only a week or two to get the job done. The sheer volume precludes doing it right.... Jack wrote of parents admonishing their children, "Go inside, kids, John's spraying." It's far past time that the DNR Environmental Protection Division start monitoring and reporting ambient levels of farm chemicals in the air. People need to know when to stay indoors.

Almost exactly one year after "We Live and Die by Chemical Agriculture" appeared in the opinion pages of the *Des Moines Register* the issue of pesticide drift was raised in the State Senate

Agriculture Committee, and yet none of the bills attempting to regulate pesticide use were allowed to make it to a floor vote. Meanwhile, the *Register* reported that about nine out of ten, or 89.6 percent, of Iowa pre-kindergarten-through-12th grade school buildings were within two thousand feet of cropland, a distance within which a 2006 National Institutes of Health study found an increased risk of potentially harmful pesticide spray drifts.

A timely op-ed could begin a wider discussion, or spearhead a larger grassroots campaign, but it could not in and of itself overcome powerful commercial interests and deeply entrenched legislative lobbies.

As I began the process of compiling and editing these pieces for publication in 2019, nearly ten years had passed. And as I reflected back on the previous decade I realized how much agriculture had diversified in practice. For example, as I traveled around the country researching my 2012 book *The Midwest Farmer's Daughter: In Search of an American Icon* I met a dynamic mix of urban farmers, woman farmers, seed-savers, and scientists working on developing perennial grains to feed a hungry world in a sustainable, environmentally-friendly fashion. In 2016 I traveled across the nation again, conducting interviews and site visits with young back-to-the-landers and Brain Drain and Brain Gain migrators for my 2017 book *Wish You Were Here: Love and Longing in an American Heartland*. Once again, I found a diversity of thought and feeling and motivation that provided solace on the otherwise lonesome roads.

The year 2020 marks an important yet unheralded centennial in America. In 1920, for the first time in history, the number of urban Americans, some 54 million, topped the number of rural Americans at just under 52 million. For one hundred years running, rural and small-town Americans have been a demographic outlier. And yet for most of that century the stock of agriculture and agriculturalists remained high in the eyes of a rapidly urbanizing nation.

As late as 2000, when I began editing my first anthology of essays on rural life, *Black Earth and Ivory Tower*, agrarians enjoyed an enduringly fine reputation, as I learned when I reached out to collaborate with Dana Hoag, a professor of agricultural economics at Colorado State University. Circa the late 1990s Hoag's research demonstrated that the basic assumptions about rural virtue had endured since Thomas Jefferson's veneration of the agrarian two-hundred years earlier. Hoag recited Jefferson's letter to John Jay from August of 1785, wherein Jefferson opined, "Cultivators of the earth are the most valuable citizens. They are the most vigorous, the most independent, the most virtuous, and they are tied to their country and wedded to its liberty and interests by the most lasting bonds."

This very belief system, Hoag assured me back then, had been kept alive by a majority in the United States who, his field research showed, continued to feel that farming was a way of life as much as a business; that it was better for a family to own a farm than a corporation; and that farmers should be their own bosses. Most people still considered agrarians more ethical, more honest, and harder working. Those same feelings led people to view farm property rights as more sacred than others, and to conclude that farmers should be protected with government subsidies or by exemptions from rules regulating conventional businesses.

In early 2011 my local Farm Bureau office asked if they might sponsor me to attend the organization's Young Farmer Conference. I was a fourth-generation member of the Bureau, a long-running affiliation begun by my great-grandfather, a farmer-writer who had not only served as an officer in the organization but had also hosted many of its local events on our farm. Initially, I demurred. I wasn't a full-fledged farmer, I pointed out with the characteristic aversion to would-bes and wanna-bes that rural people naturally develop.

Many of the break-out sessions that weekend featured a new generation of bloggers who had taken to the internet in an attempt to explain a badly misinterpreted way of life. Many had married into farm or ranch life, and still they felt a righteous indignation at the misrepresentations of rural living perpetuated by the metropolitan media. In workshop after workshop we the young farmers, agrarian writers and journalists, agricultural educators, rural policymakers, and food producers were reminded that at no time in American history were our voices needed more urgently than now.

Given time I began to think maybe the organization was right: maybe the fabled silence of the farm seen from a distance—from highway, interstate, airplane—is precisely the problem. How can the *culture* in agriculture expect to thrive if it doesn't have the time, inclination, or ability to speak its values? Perhaps we think we shouldn't need to speak our beliefs—beliefs that were once understood when farms, rather than financial services and advanced manufacturing, dominated economies in so-called farm states. Because most agrarians regard actions-speak-louder-than-words as holy writ, we have neglected to speak our truth in the websites, radio and television broadcasts, films, books, newspapers, and magazines that so loudly serve the interests of others.

One takeaway from the Young Farmer conference rang clear: younger agrarians are far more diverse politically, ideologically, and professionally than ever before. Why not let the rest of the world in on that little secret? But there were warning signs, too. While the release of the once-every-five-years Agriculture Census in 2012 prompted a surfeit of media coverage fretting over the 20 percent drop in farmers under the age of 25, that media blitz was followed by a deeper media silence. Halfway through the decade conventional commodity farming and farmers had all but disappeared from the headlines in the nation's newspapers of record.

As the decade came to a close I realized that I was a part of an ever-shrinking minority of agrarian professors. For many millennials a farm was a foreign place. Meanwhile, for many members of Generation Z "farm" had come to connote something undesirable, conflated as it was with whiteness, with landed entitlement, with patriarchy. While none of these associations applied to me or to my upbringing, I felt guilty by association, as did many farmers, ranchers, and food producers.

Still, for all the cultural downgrading of the words "farmer," "farm," or "rural," students showed more interest than ever in issues reflecting the cornerstones of agrarian thought. On my campus and on others popular academic minors and majors in environmental studies programs were introduced. Organic produce found its way into dining halls, and community gardens sunk roots in seldom-used corners of campus. Interdisciplinary seminars on food safety, food security, and fair trade became popular first-year offerings. An increasing number of students now identified as First Generation, an umbrella that included many young agrarians. First Gen's well-documented struggles with self-confidence, with persistence, and with familial support for higher education aspirations spoke to the plight of many young people raised on the land.

Over the decade in which the preceding columns and commentaries were percolating, I reached out to many scholars in agricultural history looking for kindred souls within academe, only to find that several of the most noted scholars in the field were no longer actively researching and writing the subject, moving on, apparently, to greener pastures and more fertile scholarly ground. I marveled at the matter-of-factness of their disavowals. How could one simply shed a lifetime of research in a subject area to conform to academic trends?

Though the breadth of my own scholarly and creative passions have at times taken me away from agricultural and agrarian writing, I don't believe I will ever stop writing about country views and the people who believe in them, so deeply has the agrarian life left its imprint on me. I do not seek to "graduate" from the animating force that for so long has shaped my writing and given it substance. While ten years from now I expect my voice will have evolved and transformed, just as agriculture itself will have evolved and transformed, I expect always to hear in it the voice of a faithful farmer's son.

I know too that the complex world the members of Generation Z stand ready to inherit needs experienced agrarian minds more than ever, and I fear such wisdoms will be in short supply. As the likes of Wendell Berry, Wes Jackson, and Victor Davis Hanson age and eventually pass from the green fields of this world to the greener fields beyond in years to come, the chain of farm-raised public intellectuals, teachers, educators, and researchers risks being broken, along with the intellectual and spiritual inheritance that allows a rising generation to embrace a country view of the world.

The coming decade is an ideal time, then, to build bridges to the future, renewing and refreshing the agrarian wellspring that animates our nation, feeding it, watering it, and giving it new life. Thinking back, much of my late father's advice was at root an exhortation toward gratitude. "Keep on the sunny side," he would say, echoing the hopeful bluegrass lyric from simpler times, and sometimes, "Better than to be pushing up daisies."

I am grateful, in the end, to count myself among the living, like the red-winged blackbirds that ride the husks of reeds each spring full of words and chatter, full of opinions large and small, of complaints and blessings, of lamentations and love—of life itself.

Acknowledgments

"Portrait of a Harvest," "Angling for Amazon," "In Praise of Barnyard English," "We're Dying Here," "Homecoming Redo," "Rural Ghouls," "Cyber Monday in the Country," "Holidays on Ice," "New Crops and Old Worries," "Seasonal Disaffections," and "Mind of Winter" first appeared in the *Daily Yonder*, some under alternate title. © Zachary Michael Jack 2013–2017.

"When High-Speed internet Comes to the Slow Lane," "A Man Among Marching Women," "We Live and Die by Chemical Agriculture," and "Our Ancestors Sleep Down the Road" first appeared in the *Des Moines Register*, © Zachary Michael Jack 2015–2017.

"Last Man Standing," "Father's Day and a Film that Gets Rural America Right," "Too Old to Rock and Roll, Young Enough to Protest," "A Time for Cheering" "Barefoot Eras" and "Autumnal Swings" first appeared, under alternate title, in the *Iowa Source*. © Zachary Michael Jack 2008–2014.

"The Rural Health Care Crisis Is Real" first appeared in the *Waterloo-Cedar Falls Courier* under the title "The Midwest's Rural Health Care Crisis is Real." © Zachary Michael Jack 2017.

"Twilight-time: An Open Letter" appeared under alternate title and in different form in *Letters to a Young Iowan*. © Zachary Michael Jack, 2007.

"Mothers' Day," "Savoring Straw Polls," and "Moving Beyond 'It Could Have Been Worse'" first appeared in the *Cedar Rapids Gazette* under the titles "Three Cheers for Grandmothers on Mother's Day" and "In Defense of the Iowa Straw Poll" and "More Than the Sum of Our Natural Disasters." © Zachary Michael Jack 2015–2017.

"Agrarian Fireworks" first appeared in *Front Porch Republic*. © Zachary Michael Jack 2016.

"The Red Glow of Pyrotechnic Shifts" first appeared in the *Quad City Times* under the title "Are Fireworks a Harbinger for Shifting Politics?" © Zachary Michael Jack 2017.

"The Plot of Grassroots Politics" first appeared, in alternate form, under the title "Political Imagination and the Campaign Narrative in the journal *Pro Rege*, Volume 44, Number 3. © Zachary Michael Jack 2016.

"Family Business Not Necessarily Nepotism" first appeared in the *St. Joseph News-Press*. © Zachary Michael Jack 2017.

"A Rural Rip Van Winkle" first appeared under the title "Rip Van Winkle Was a Man" in *The Good Men Project*. © Zachary Michael Jack 2016.

About the Author

Zachary Michael Jack's columns and commentaries have appeared in many of the nation's best-circulated newspapers, from *USA Today* and the *Los Angeles Times*, to the *San Francisco Chronicle*, to the *Milwaukee Journal-Sentinel* and the *Albuquerque Journal*. A one-time newspaper section editor, Jack has written many books on rural history and culture, earning multiple nominations for the Theodore Saloutos Award for the year's best book on agriculture. Jack's most recent title on agrarian life and the power of place is *Wish You Were Here: Love and Longing in an American Heartland*. He is a member of the national board of directors for the Midwestern History Association (MHA) and serves on the faculty of the Writing and Chicago Area Studies programs at North Central College in Naperville, Illinois, where he teaches courses in writing for social change and place studies, among others. Jack is a seventh-generation rural Iowan.

About the Imprint: What makes a book a Tall Corn Book? A scholarly or creative focus on the culture of Iowa, the Tall Corn State, and the surrounding region written by well-established authors celebrating the unique cultures and contributions of the land where corn is king.

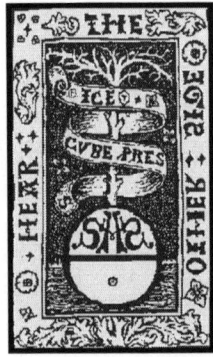

The Ice Cube Press began publishing in 1991 to focus on how to live with the natural world and to better understand how people can best live together in the communities they share and inhabit. Using the literary arts to explore life and experiences in the heartland of the United States we have been recognized by a number of well-known writers including: Gary Snyder, Gene Logsdon, Wes Jackson, Patricia Hampl, Greg Brown, Jim Harrison, Annie Dillard, Ken Burns, Roz Chast, Jane Hamilton, Daniel Menaker, Kathleen Norris, Janisse Ray, Craig Lesley, Alison Deming, Harriet Lerner, Richard Lynn Stegner, Richard Rhodes, Michael Pollan, David Abram, David Orr, and Barry Lopez. We've published a number of well-known authors including: Mary Swander, Jim Heynen, Mary Pipher, Bill Holm, Connie Mutel, John T. Price, Carol Bly, Marvin Bell, Debra Marquart, Ted Kooser, Stephanie Mills, Bill McKibben, Craig Lesley, Elizabeth McCracken, Derrick Jensen, Dean Bakopoulos, Rick Bass, Linda Hogan, Pam Houston, and Paul Gruchow. Check out Ice Cube Press books on our web site, join our email list, Facebook group, or follow us on Twitter. Visit booksellers, museum shops, or any place you can find good books and support true honest to goodness independent publishing projects so you can discover why we continue striving to "hear the other side."

Ice Cube Press, LLC (Est. 1991)
North Liberty, Iowa, Midwest, USA
steve@icecubepress.com
twitter @icecubepress
www.IceCubePress.com

To Fenna Marie
A beautiful and loving
daughter, growing up
in the heartland